Surfing the

A Novel way to Cope With Food Cravings

Educational and therapeutic pages for
you to ponder, color and embellish.

Created by:

Sarah A. Moore, Registered Dietitian, Yoga Teacher and Board Certified
Specialist in Obesity and Weight management

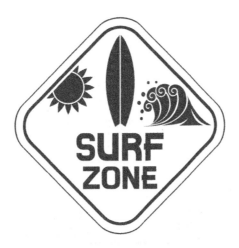

These are my original words and images created and modified with Canva, Inkscape and Midjourney

For more inspiration and to heal your relationship with food check out:
www.RisingNutrition.com

Dedication Page

This activity book is a heartfelt dedication to everyone who has trusted me to help them heal their relationship with food. It's also an invitation to those I haven't yet worked with, offering a chance to improve their relationship with themselves and food. Through the use of color, mindfulness, creativity, and journaling, I invite you to embark on an empowering journey of crafting a healthy food story using your imagination.

Years ago, my high school pottery teacher introduced me to the concept that "art heals." This guidance has shaped my life positively. I've used art to process, cope with, and heal from many of life's challenges. If you're already using art and imagination to heal, I applaud you. If not, consider this your personal invitation to start.

Coloring can help manage anxiety and improve mood, making it a valuable tool when changing eating habits causes stress. Use this activity book as an anchor to ground yourself and as a surfboard to stay afloat when you feel overwhelmed.

Within these pages, you'll discover inspiration, guidance, and tools to reshape your narrative around food. Start fostering a nourishing and fulfilling connection with yourself and the food that sustains you.

Also, I want to say congratulations on taking the first step toward a healthier you by turning inspiration into action and beginning to work through this book. If you are looking to take things a step further, visit www.RisingNutrition.com and contact me or scan the QR code below and color along with me on YouTube as I reflect on concepts in this book, my own journey with food and self-image and help guide you through yours.

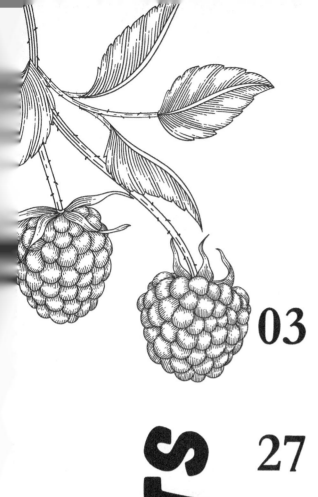

TABLE OF CONTENTS

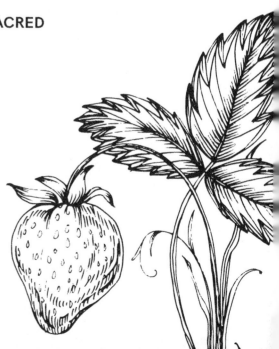

Introduction

Dear Eater,

As I reflect on the challenge of dealing with unwanted food cravings faced by both my patients and myself, I ponder this question: "How can I offer a more profound and creative solution?" In the midst of this contemplation, I drifted off to sleep, only to awaken at 3 a.m. with a brilliant idea: an adult coloring book. I couldn't contain my excitement and immediately jotted the idea down in my journal. Over the following week, it became clear that many of us crave tangible tools to help manage our food cravings and heal our relationship with food.

And so, the concept of "Surfing the Urge" was born. Fortunately, I had my trusty sketchbook and colored pencils at hand! I eagerly set to work on creating the pages of the workbook that now rests in your hands. From my perspective as a dietitian, I firmly believe that food can serve as a nurturing sanctuary, a refuge during emotional storms, a moment for refueling, and an opportunity for quiet introspection, allowing us to reclaim our personal power. It is during these times that we acknowledge that our soul not only resides within us but also has a place at the table.

Through years of providing medical nutrition therapy to individuals navigating the complexities of our modern food world and confronting my own food-related challenges, I have come to realize that the power of nourishment has been wrested from our grasp. It has been commandeered by industry, science, and the media. Our food choices are often driven by ingrained habits, addiction to hyperpalatable foods, incessant marketing campaigns, and obsessive thoughts regarding what we should or should not consume. We have lost sight of why we eat and the true purpose food can serve.

If you are reading this, it signifies your desire to reclaim your personal food narrative and mend your relationship with food, transforming it from a source of stress to one of sustenance.

This workbook will serve as your guide in navigating the treacherous waters of cravings. We will employ evidence-based strategies rooted in nutritional, psychological, and spiritual concepts. While the creative presentation of some of these concepts may be novel, many of the strategies are familiar and proven. At the conclusion of this book, you will find a list of resources to further support your journey. As well as information to download a free bonus chapter.

Now is the time to embrace the practice of slowing down, granting yourself the luxury of nourishment and self-connection.

Welcome to the next level of mindful eating.

Sincerely,
Sarah A. Moore, RDN, CSOWM, CYT

COLOR PALLET
Color, mix, and label.

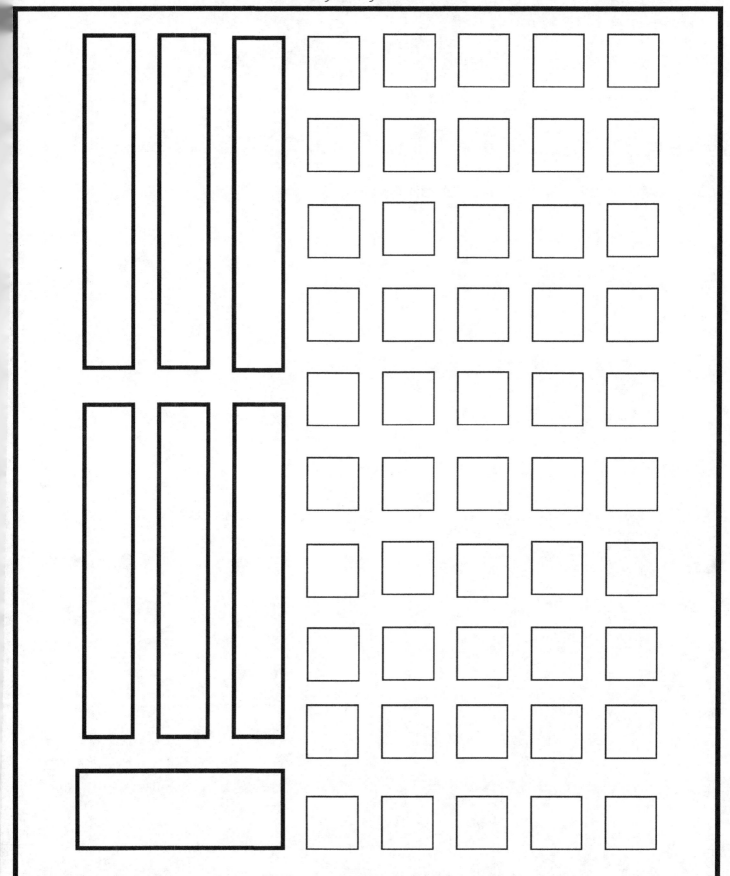

Part I
Exploring Food Cravings

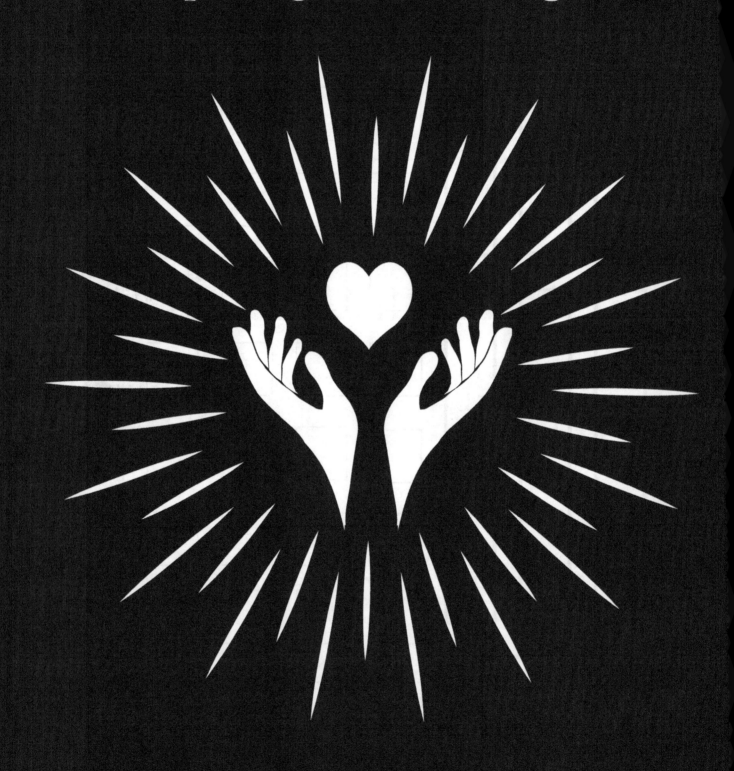

Understanding Food Cravings

What do They Mean?

Does craving fatty, oily foods indicate a need for calcium? Or, when experiencing muscle spasms, which can be a sign of magnesium deficiency, do you instinctively crave pumpkin seeds, a good source of magnesium? Current research indicates a definitive no. Even in cases of PICA, a condition involving compulsive consumption of food or non-food items linked to mineral deficiency, individuals do not typically seek out a food containing the specific nutrient they lack.

So, are food cravings solely driven by our pleasure-seeking systems? That answer is also no. The truth is more nuanced, existing within a complex, non-linear system. The neuroendocrine system, comprising hormones and the nervous system, plays a crucial role in our food cravings. Also, we may crave a food because we like a food, or because we are tired, we are in our menstrual cycle, we are anxious or depressed, our body is in need of sodium, an abundance of unfavorable bacteria in our intestines or we are in a state of insulin resistance or excess insulin production.

Deprivation

Getting caught up in food moralization, labeling certain foods as good or bad, can make us feel ashamed of liking "bad" foods. When we draw rigid lines, such as saying, "I am never going to eat this again," we create a sense of deprivation that can drive cravings. While it's true that depriving ourselves of a food we like can increase our craving for it, it's also true that the foods we crave are often a result of a conditioned response, much like a puppy trained to want its favorite treat. Interestingly, when abstinence from a desired food is chosen voluntarily, it can actually reduce our craving for that food.

Sodium

Sodium stands out as a unique nutrient in our dietary history, as it wasn't abundant in our ancestors' diets. Because of this, our bodies have adapted to prioritize sodium intake, leading to cravings when we're deficient. A lack of sodium can manifest in severe symptoms like nausea, vomiting, diarrhea, or even heat stroke, highlighting its critical role. Interestingly, our bodies can create new neural pathways to crave higher sodium levels chronically, aiming to prevent deficiency due to its significant risks. This complicates the evaluation of sodium cravings, as they can stem from neuroendocrine adaptation, hedonic pleasure, or genuine dietary deficiency.

To assess the origin of your salt cravings, conducting a sodium audit is recommended. This involves tracking your sodium intake in milligrams (mg) for three days, with the target range being 2,000 to 3,000mg daily. If your intake falls below this range, adding more salt to your diet may be necessary to reduce unwanted salt cravings. Conversely, if your intake is significantly higher, your cravings might be attributed to a heightened sensitivity and preference to sodium. Understanding the source of your sodium cravings can help you make informed dietary choices and ensure you're meeting your body's needs without overdoing it.

Sugar

In regards to sugar cravings there is a lot we still do not know, luckily researchers are diligently working to understand sugar cravings. We do know that eating sugar feeds unfavorable bacteria in the intestines and there is evidence that can continue to cause more sugar cravings. In order to nourish healthy bacteria eating complex carbohydrates and probiotic rich foods like yogurt, kimchi, sauerkraut, kombucha is essential. If you are struggling with gastrointestinal issues, it would be beneficial to see a medical professional to address it.

Additionally, there are many hormones in the body that impact our hunger and cravings. The main players in this story are insulin and glucagon. Insulin is the hormone most in charge of our sugar cravings. And, strangely enough it is the insufficient or excess production of insulin or a cellular resistance to using it that causes the metabolism to fall into chaos. The mixed up signaling causes cellular metabolism to slow down, energy storage to go up all while food cravings to go up. If you have a family history of diabetes, PCOS, fatty liver or easily put on belly fat it would be beneficial to see a medical professional and do the appropriate lab work because certain medications and supplements can bring order to the metabolic chaos.

Yet, your sugar cravings could be as simple as you are in the habit of eating dessert or maybe you succumb to the craving as an energy fix in the middle of the day. Either way, surfing the sugar craving urge is challenging but doable. And in the end, once you get off the sugar roller coaster, eat more macro balanced meals the cravings do calm down.

Menstrual Cycle

Are you craving sweets around your menstrual cycle? You're not alone, and it's not just in your head. These increased cravings are supported by science. Serotonin production greatly increases as estrogen production rises and it goes the other way as well, often he times of month when your body is low in serotonin and you need to feel happier or your body is producing a lot of it is when you feel the food tug. The increase in serotonin depends on the presence of tryptophan and insulin secretion, which is triggered by the sight and consumption of sweet foods. During these times your body will want something sweet to stimulate insulin, but what you crave is conditioned. To satisfy your cravings and support your body's natural processes, reach for fruits rich in natural sugars like berries, apples, or citrus fruits. They'll not only help curb your sweet tooth but also provide essential nutrients. So next time you feel the urge, grab a piece of fruit and enjoy the sweet taste while giving your body the nourishment it needs.

Research does indicate that people who have the diets with the lowest intake of vitamins and minerals do report high food cravings, so with that being identified it is important to ensure you are eating a variety of foods that contain all of the essential vitamins, minerals and amino acids.

Sleep

Sleep deficiency elevates the hunger hormone ghrelin in the body. Additionally, it elevates certain chemicals in the endocannabinoid system, making you not only feel hungrier but also crave higher-calorie foods with that delicious, fatty sweetness. These biochemical changes and the behavioral response have been tested and reproduced in numerous research studies. It's now somewhat common knowledge that if you want to reduce food cravings and possibly lose weight, one of the first things to do is to address the quality and duration of your sleep. Ready to make a change? Start by prioritizing your sleep!

Food Nutrient Table

Vitamin	Food Source
A	Liver, fish liver oil, dairy products, carrots, sweet potatoes
D	Fatty fish (salmon, mackerel), liver, egg yolks, fortified foods
E	Nuts, seeds, vegetable oils, olive and nut oil, leafy greens, fortified cereals
K	Leafy greens, broccoli, liver, fish, eggs
B1 (Thiamine)	Whole grains, pork, nuts, seeds
B2 (Riboflavin)	Dairy products, eggs, lean meats, green vegetables
B3 (Niacin)	Meat, fish, poultry, whole grains, mushrooms
B5 (Pantothenic Acid)	Avocado, chicken, beef, potatoes, whole grains
B6 (Pyridoxine)	Chickpeas, beef liver, tuna, salmon, potatoes
B7 (Biotin)	Eggs, nuts, sweet potatoes, spinach, mushrooms
B9 (Folate)	Leafy greens, legumes, asparagus, avocado, citrus fruits
B12 (Cobalamin)	Meat, fish, poultry, dairy products, fortified cereals
C (Ascorbic Acid)	Oranges, grapefruit, kiwi fruit, strawberries, bell peppers

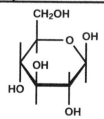

Food is Information for the Body!

Food Nutrient Table

Mineral	Food Source
Calcium	Dairy products (milk, cheese, yogurt), leafy greens, nuts, seeds
Iron	Red meat, poultry, lentils, beans, spinach, fortified cereals
Magnesium	Nuts, seeds, whole grains, leafy greens, fish, beans
Phosphorus	Dairy products, meat, poultry, fish, nuts, whole grains
Potassium	Bananas, oranges, potatoes, tomatoes, beans, dairy products
Zinc	Red meat, poultry, seafood, beans, nuts, dairy products
Selenium	Brazil nuts, fish, poultry, eggs, spinach, sunflower seeds
Copper	Shellfish, whole grains, nuts, seeds, beans, potatoes
Manganese	Nuts, seeds, whole grains, leafy greens, tea
Iodine	Seafood, dairy products, iodized salt

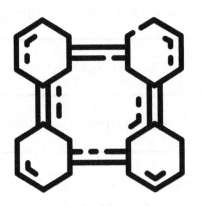

As I indicated earlier your neuroendocrine system is responsible for some of the cravings you experience, this may be related to having poor sleep and craving sweets or it may be related to the need for specific nutrients to help with neurotransmitter production. The body needs specific amino acids to create neurotransmitters and although we would like it, if the body knew what it needed and cause us to crave the specific foods containing those nutrients, once again it just doesn't work that way.

One way to address the need is to understand what food or beverage provides what specific nutrients so you ensure you consume them. The amino acids below are all associated with mood and energy regulation. If you find that you lose focus in the afternoon are depressed or have trouble falling asleep these foods can nourish those systems and ultimately help reduce cravings or at least guide you in the direction of nourishing consumption.

Foods to Nourish Healthy Neurotransmitters and Help With Energy and Mood	
Foods that increase GABA Levels	Fermented foods (kimchi, sauerkraut, miso, tempeh), Whole grains (oats, barley, buckwheat, brown rice), soy products (tofu, tempeh) Fish (mackerel, halibut, shrimp) Nuts and seeds (almonds, walnuts, sunflower seeds, pumpkin seeds, chia seeds) Cruciferous Vegetables (Broccoli, cauliflower, brussel sprouts, cabbage, kale, bok choy, arugula, collard green, radishes, turnips) Tea (green tea, black tea), cocoa (dark chocolate)
Food Sources of L-theanine	Matcha, green tea, black tea, white tea Bay Bolete mushrooms Some types of green algae
Food Sources of Tryptophan	Turkey, chicken, pork, fish (salmon, halibut, tuna) Eggs, dairy products (milk, cheese, yogurt) Nuts and seeds (pumpkin, sesame, sunflower), legumes (beans, lentils, chickpeas) Tofu and soy products, oats, banana
Food Sources of Glutamine	Beef, chicken, fish, dairy products, eggs, cabbage, spinach, beans and legumes, nuts and seeds, whole grains
Food Sources of Tyrosine	Meat, fish, dairy products, eggs, nuts and seeds, beans and legumes, soy products, whole grains, avocado, banana
Food Sources of L-Phenylalanine	Meat, fish, dairy products, eggs, nuts and seeds, beans and legumes, soy products, whole grains, vegetables (spinach, kale, broccoli), fruits (bananas, apples)

Food Cravings & Our Enriched Food Environment

The reality is that although some of our food cravings are biologically driven, not all of them. Many do come from learned experience, nostalgia, perceived value and environmental exposure. All too often I will have clients express their struggle watching TV simply because the number of food related commercials, I can promise they are not alone in their struggle nor is it just their impression. The literature consistently shows that both food and drug cues can significantly increase craving. Studies have demonstrated that exposure to drug-related stimuli leads to a marked increase in self-reported craving across various substances of abuse. Similarly, exposure to food cues has been shown to significantly enhance craving for food. Importantly, research indicates that exposure to food cues not only triggers physiological responses and craving but also results in increased eating behavior. Additionally, the extent of cue reactivity and cue-induced craving has been found to consistently predict subsequent eating and weight gain in both adults and children.

A recent meta-analysis systematically examined the effects of food cue exposure, cue reactivity, and craving on eating and weight-related outcomes in both the short- and long-term. The analysis suggested that food exposure and craving play a significant role in promoting eating and weight gain. These findings support the notion that food cues can stimulate craving, leading to increased insulin which results in increased hunger and eventually eating. Another meta-analysis focusing on studies using food advertisements as cues found a small-to-moderate effect size, indicating that exposure to food advertising is associated with increased eating. Together, these studies highlight the influence of the simple notion that the more abundant the exposure is of food, the more likely we are to crave a food and that suggests that craving plays a crucial role in driving consumption and thus potentially weight gain.

Not only can environmental cues from processed, highly palatable foods containing the perfect blend of salt, sugar, and fat cause us to eat more and gain weight, but they can also become addictive substances. Multiple studies on humans and animals have shown that items like table sugar, saccharin, ice cream, candy, soda, and other processed foods trigger addictive behaviors such as loss of control, inability to stop eating, and impaired impulse control. If you think you may be struggling with food addiction, continue working through this book and seek a health professional to discuss the topic. There are also food addiction support groups online and rehab facilities that can help.

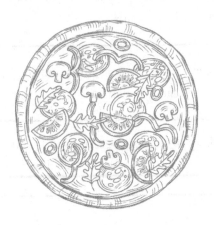

Intensity of the Heat

Eating plays a vital role in regulating our mood, energy, and cognitive function. It's no surprise, then, that during moments of emotional overwhelm, we often turn to food for comfort and distraction. However, when relying on food becomes an unwanted coping mechanism, it's important to explore alternative strategies. Nevertheless, it's essential to acknowledge that food can still be a part of our story. The approach I propose has proven effective for both my clients and myself. One helpful tool is the "emotional overwhelm thermometer" to determine whether it's an appropriate time to use food as a coping mechanism:

Step 1: Recall a recent mildly stressful situation and note the corresponding physical sensations on the thermometer at 25%. Repeat this exercise for 50%, 75%, and 100% stress levels. This process will help you gauge your current stress level and better understand your emotional state.

Step 2: When experiencing emotions that are at or below the 75% mark on the emotional overwhelm thermometer, it's important to challenge the urge to engage in stress eating. Instead, focus on practicing the art of surfing the urge. However, if the stress level exceeds 75%, it's okay to give yourself permission to eat. The key is to shift gears and approach eating mindfully, paying attention to the sensations and experiences associated with the food.

If you notice that numerous small stressors are accumulating and pushing you into the 75-100% zone, it's crucial to address the underlying reasons behind these triggers. Taking the time to understand and tackle these smaller stressors can help prevent them from accumulating and overwhelming you.

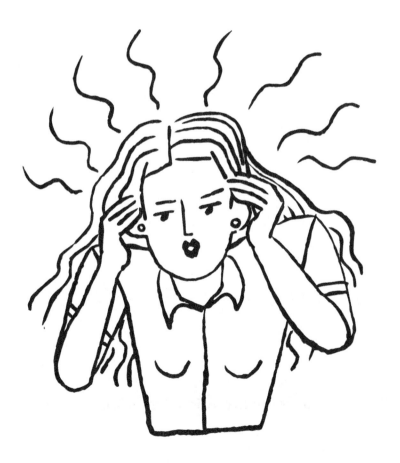

This Page Intentionally Left Blank

Intensity of the Heat

In Practice

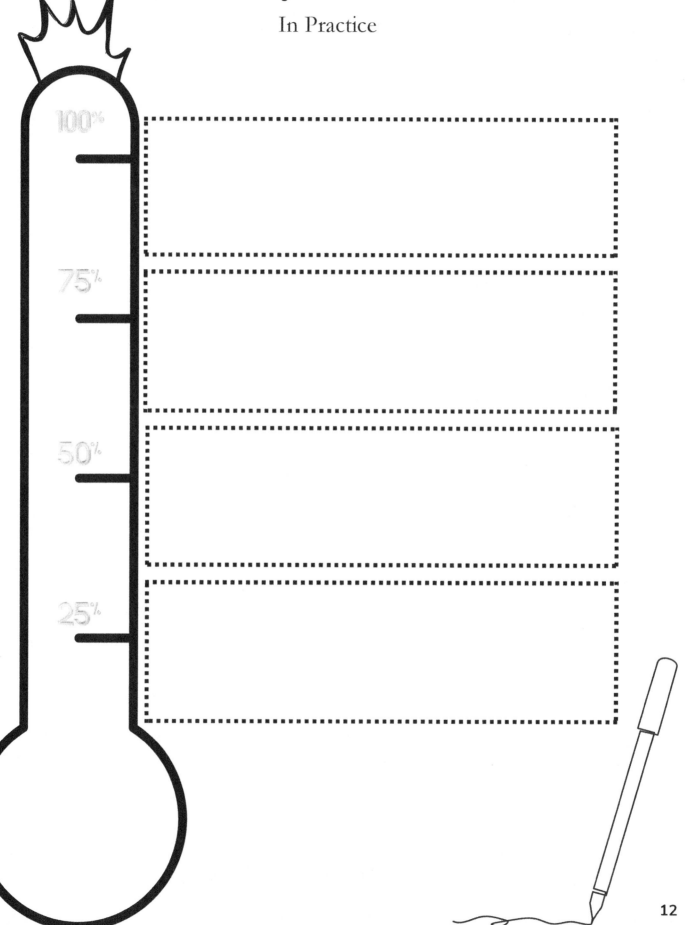

Food for Good Mood and Energy

Having worked with thousands of people to improve the way they eat, cravings and stress eating always come up as a topic. And before I assume the issue is purely behavioral I always focus in on how their meals or lack of meals are impacting their body on a deeper biological level.

In order to properly nourish our body there are three simple concepts to keep in mind: timing, amount and balance. If we don't have the right timing, amount and balance at meals it will cause us to excessively crave foods, feel highs and lows in our energy or possibly not even hungry all day until the evening and then we can't stop grazing throughout the evening.

Timing of our meals impacts our blood sugar, metabolic rate and how energized we feel. When we go long periods of time without eating our body breaks down glycogen into glucose (sugar) that is released into our blood stream. When this glucose is released into our blood stream it requires insulin to facilitate using that fuel efficiently. If we have insulin resistance or insufficient or excessive insulin production we will end up with big swings in our blood sugar. Those big swings in blood sugar impact our mood and energy, thus impacting our cravings for foods that increase our mood or energy (caffeine and carbs!).

Amount of food, each specific (macronutrient), fiber, micronutrients at a meal impact how satiating it will be to our body. It takes about 15 minutes for a glass of juice to be digested and absorbed, an orange will take about 60 minutes but something like a piece of chicken thigh will take 2-4 hours and an avocado more like 4-6. Carbohydrates digest the quickest, protein next and fat is the slowest. The total amount and type of food impacts how long we are satisfied.

This leads into our next point, balance. Balanced amount of protein, carbohydrate and fat at a meal impacts our blood sugar and energy. When the balance at the meal is dominated by simple sugar or starchy carbohydrates we digest quicker with more blood sugar variability and end up with more cravings for food to regulate (yes you guessed it) our mood and energy.

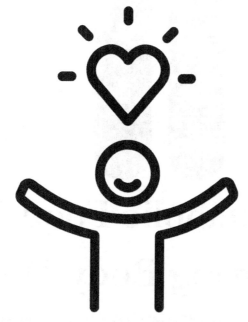

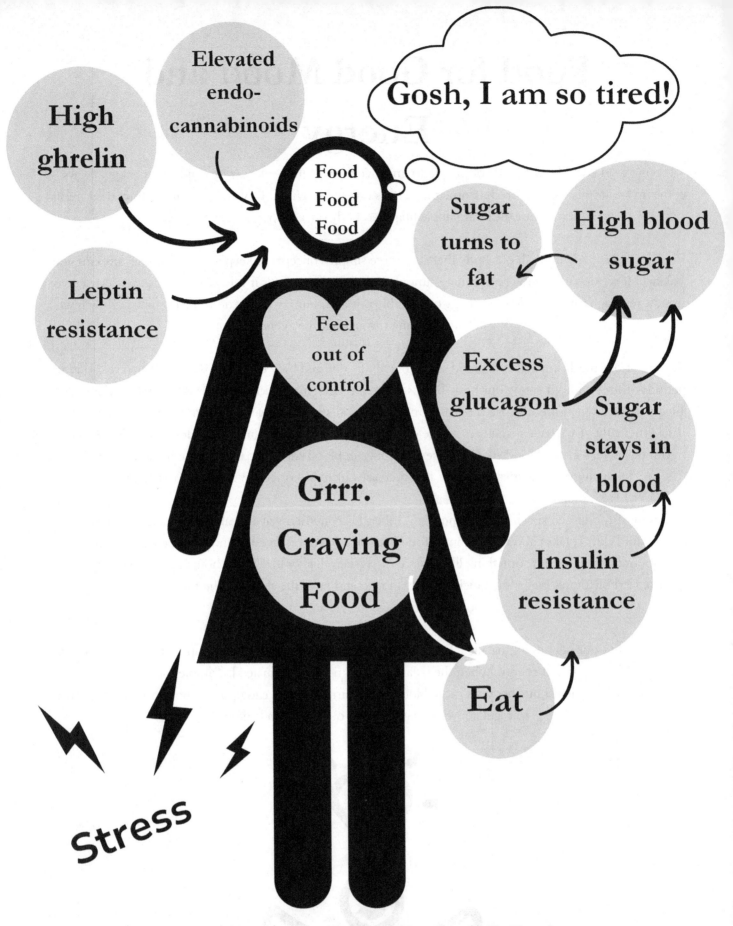

What is Your Personal Profile

Describe the Experience in Your Body

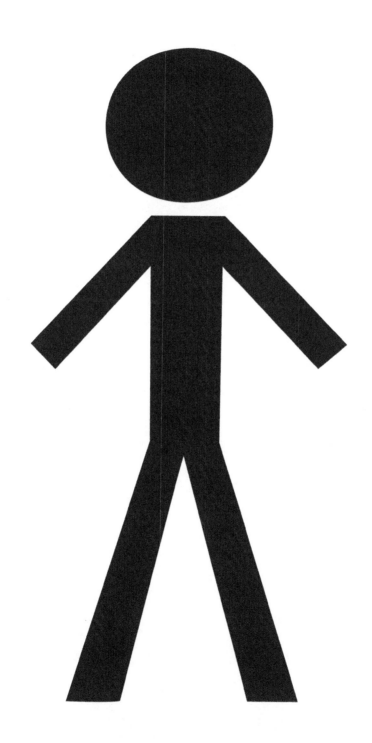

Choose to Eat Mindfully

To begin eating mindfully, it is crucial to grasp the concept of mindless eating, as researched by Brian Wansink, PhD. This concept reveals how subtle environmental factors can lead us to overeat without awareness. For instance, large portions served at restaurants, driving past a fast food restaurant, big plates, or having food in plain sight can all contribute to mindless overeating. In addition to the many external cues that can lead to mindless eating, there are also internal cues that are often unconscious. These include eating for emotional regulation, eating out of habit, eating due to boredom, fear of not having food in the future, eating to fit into a social situation, and not tuning into one's senses. Which are the episodes of eating we are learning to surf. In these situations that we often tend tune out and the antidote is to tune in. As we begin to learn that these episodes are not as fulfilling the likeliness that they stop happening increases. By recognizing these influences, we can make more conscious choices. Becoming aware of the reward and Mindful eating is about being aware and intentional with our actions, fully present with our senses. It is not about *not wanting cake*. It is about tuning into our five senses—sight, sound, smell, touch, and taste—when we sit down to eat.

When we eat mindfully, we observe, describe, act with awareness, and maintain a nonjudgmental and nonreactive attitude toward our eating experience. From this place, we have both feet on the ground in reality, making mindful eating a empowering practice. By eating mindfully we can begin to take smaller bites, chew our food well and truly savor the pleasure and nourishment it provides.

To begin eating mindfully, consider these questions:

What environmental factors might be influencing your eating habits?

How can you make your eating environment more conducive to mindful eating, such as turning off the TV?

Can you identify any mindless eating moments in your daily life?

Is there any way to make them mindful, could eating with chopsticks help slow your pace of eating?

Are judgements about food getting in the way of being present when I eat?

What small changes can you make to become more aware and intentional with your eating?

Would it be possible to use a smaller bowl or plate and dish up less food, to see if your physical hunger was fulfilled with less?

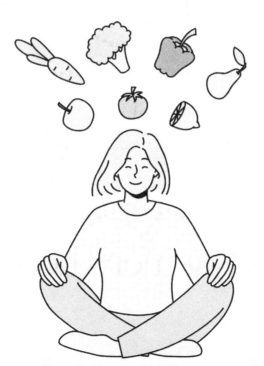

This Acknowledges

THAT

YOUR NAME HERE

RECEIVES THIS

CERTIFICATE OF ACHIEVEMENT

FOR NO LONGER WANTING CAKE!

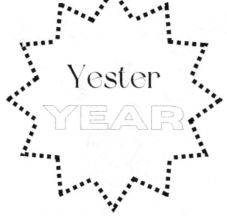

Yester
YEAR

Food Shamers League

My Macronutrients

Protein

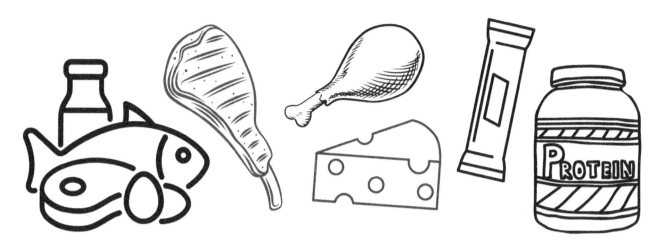

Carbohydrates

Fat

This Page Intentionally Left Blank

Carbohydrates have two categories:

Starchy

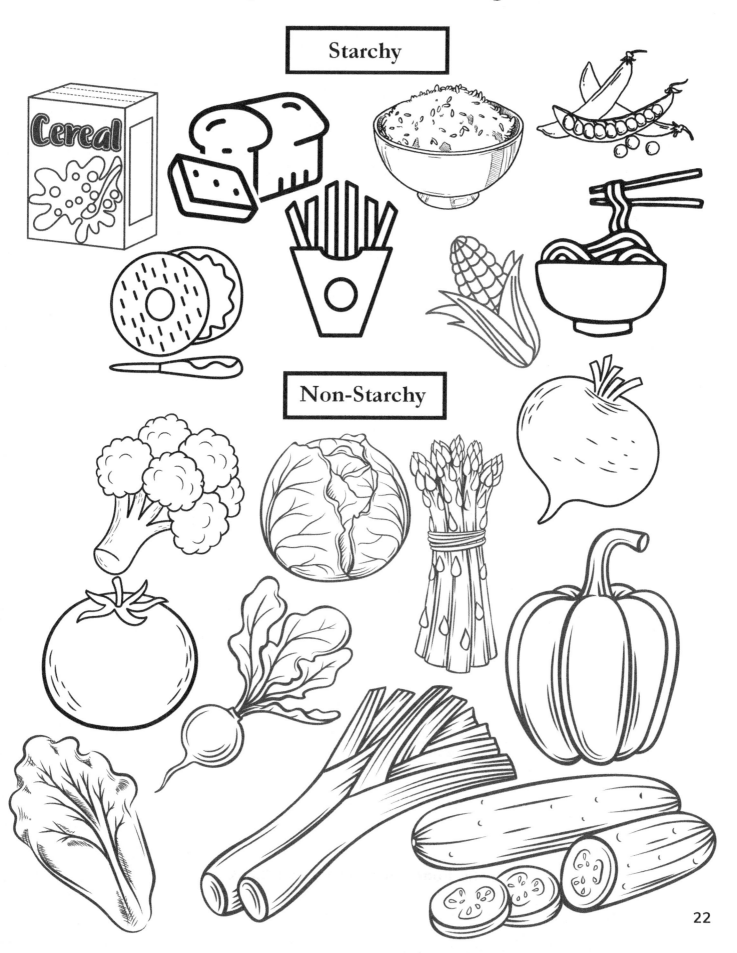

Non-Starchy

This Page Intentionally Left Blank

Sample Meal Plan

For stable energy and blood sugar include all all macronutrients at a meal or pair carbohydrates with protein and/or fat.

Breakfast

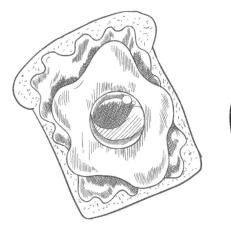
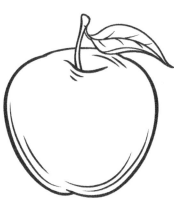
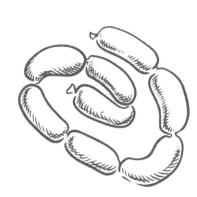

Lunch

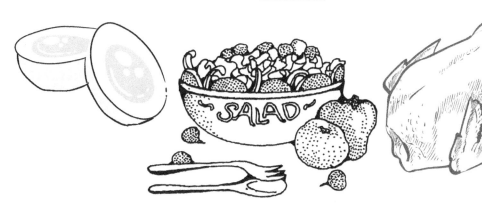

Dinner

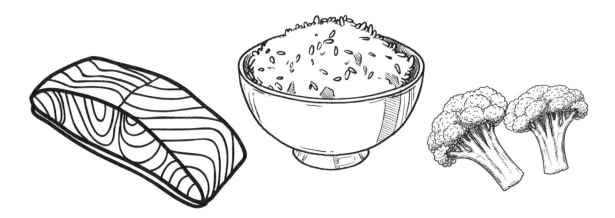

This Page Intentionally Left Blank

Sample Vegetarian Meal Plan

Breakfast

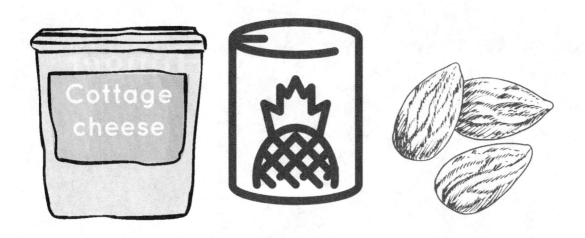

Lunch

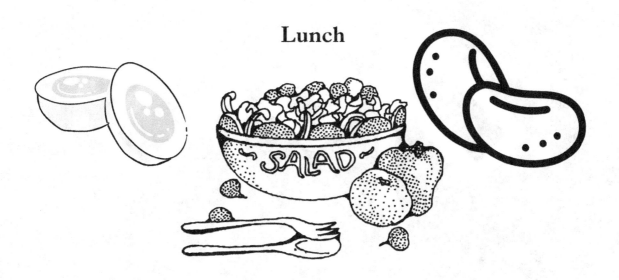

Dinner

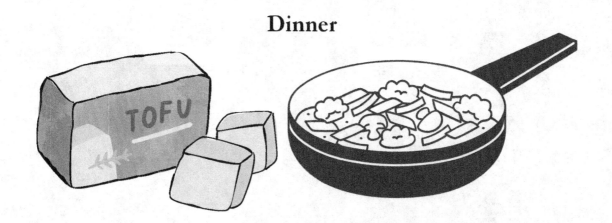

Part II

Getting to Know Hunger

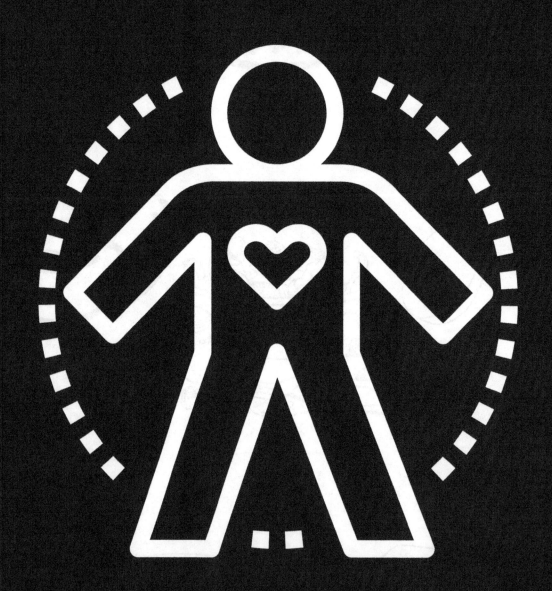

Hunger

Frequently, my patients share thoughts like, "I'd be so much healthier if I didn't crave _____," referencing their love for specific foods. As humans, we relish the taste of good food, whether sweet or savory. Despite this, we often feel guilty for indulging in our favorite treats, even though it's entirely normal to crave them. The nutrition propaganda machine has convinced us that liking, craving, or eating certain foods is somehow wrong, but it's time to redefine our relationship with food. This involves exploring the what, when, and why of the foods we choose or choose not to eat, which can be uncomfortable and scary. Importantly, having a positive relationship with food doesn't mean removing emotions from eating or viewing food solely as fuel. Instead, it means being informed and empowered to consciously nourish our bodies and enjoy the pleasure food provides.

In order to understanding our relationship with food, it's crucial to recognize the different types of hunger we experience. Physical hunger is the biological need for food and arises when our body requires energy. Mental hunger, on the other hand, occurs when we crave food based on external cues like seeing an advertisement or smelling something delicious. Finally, emotional hunger emerges when we use food as a coping mechanism to deal with stress, boredom, or other emotions. By identifying and addressing these different types of hunger, we can learn to nourish ourselves in a way that is both physically and emotionally fulfilling. This chapter will assist you in recognizing and differentiating between these types of hunger so that you can make mindful choices when it comes to your what, when and how you eat.

Do you often find yourself unsure if you're genuinely hungry or just eating out of boredom or emotional distress? Struggling to distinguish between different types of hunger, such as physical hunger, mental hunger, and emotional hunger, is a common challenge. If this sounds familiar, you're not alone. Many people grapple with recognizing and addressing their various hunger cues, leading to overeating and unhealthy food choices. In this chapter you will find a quiz has been developed to help you identify your primary type of hunger, understand its underlying causes, and learn how to nourish yourself effectively. One of the reasons we may struggle to understand what type of hunger we are feeling is because we may have different body signals for hunger and fullness than we were taught or are aware of. Below is a word find with a variety of terms used to describe hunger and fullness. What terms resonate for you and why?

```
E H Q B E W R U M B L I N G S
P O L H M A E F A H V G R T A
C L I S P T C A C E G R N I T
O L G S T E O T H A V O A G I
L O H H Y R N I E D H W U H S
D W T A G Y T G H A I L S T F
R K H K N M E U E C C I E N I
P S E I A O N E A H C N O E E
L T A N W U T D V E U G U S D
E U D E I T G Z Y V P Y S S P
A F E S N H F U L L S W N L A
S F D S G R U N N Y N O S E N
E E S S T A R V E D W E A K G
D D H A N G R Y B L O A T E D
B P E I R R I T A B L E T R T
```

Light headed	Hiccups
Shakiness	Empty
Rumbling	Irritable
Headache	Growling
Bloated	Fatigued
Heavy	Nauseous
Pleased	Stuffed
Hangry	Tightness
Watery mouth	Hollow
Satisfied	Weak
Runny nose	Cold
Gnawing	Ache
Starved	Pang
Content	Full

Hunger Quiz

	Yes	No
1. Did you eat breakfast today?	☐	☐
2. Has it been longer than 4 hours since your last meal?	☐	☐
3. Are you feeling weakness or fatigue?	☐	☐
4. Are you feeling nausea?	☐	☐
5. Did you see something that made you think of eating?	☐	☐
6. Is this food sitting on the counter or within your line of sight?	☐	☐
7. Are you craving this food?	☐	☐
8. Are you feeling bored?	☐	☐
9. Are you tired or burnt out?	☐	☐
10. Are you feeling sad, upset, angry or frustrated?	☐	☐
11. Are you feeling nervous or anxious?	☐	☐
12. Are you celebrating something?	☐	☐

If you answered yes to questions 1-4, then you are likely hungry for physical reasons.

If you answered yes to questions 5-7, then you are likely hungry for mental or habit based reasons.

If you answered yes to questions 8-12, then you are likely hungry for emotional reasons, whether this is to enhance or detract from a feeling.

If you answered yes to a variety of questions, then it is likely you are physically hungry, feeling emotional and choosing what to eat out of habit.

What is something you learned about yourself ?

Can you take action on that? If so, what would you do?

Physical Hunger

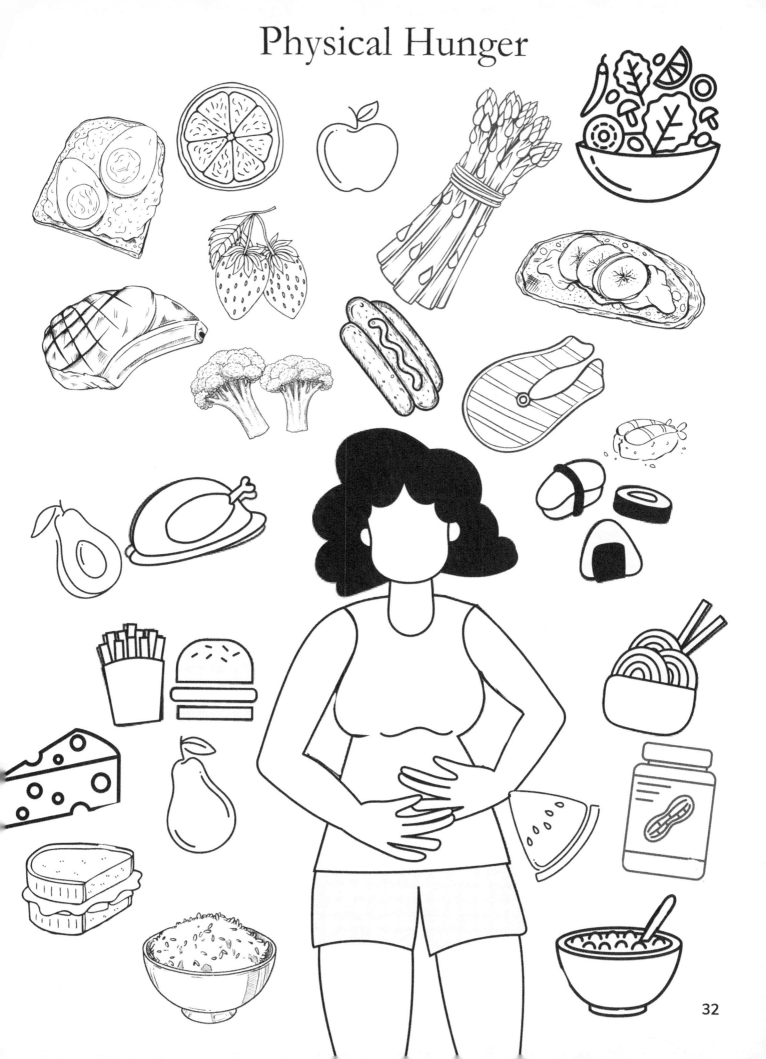

This Page Intentionally Left Blank

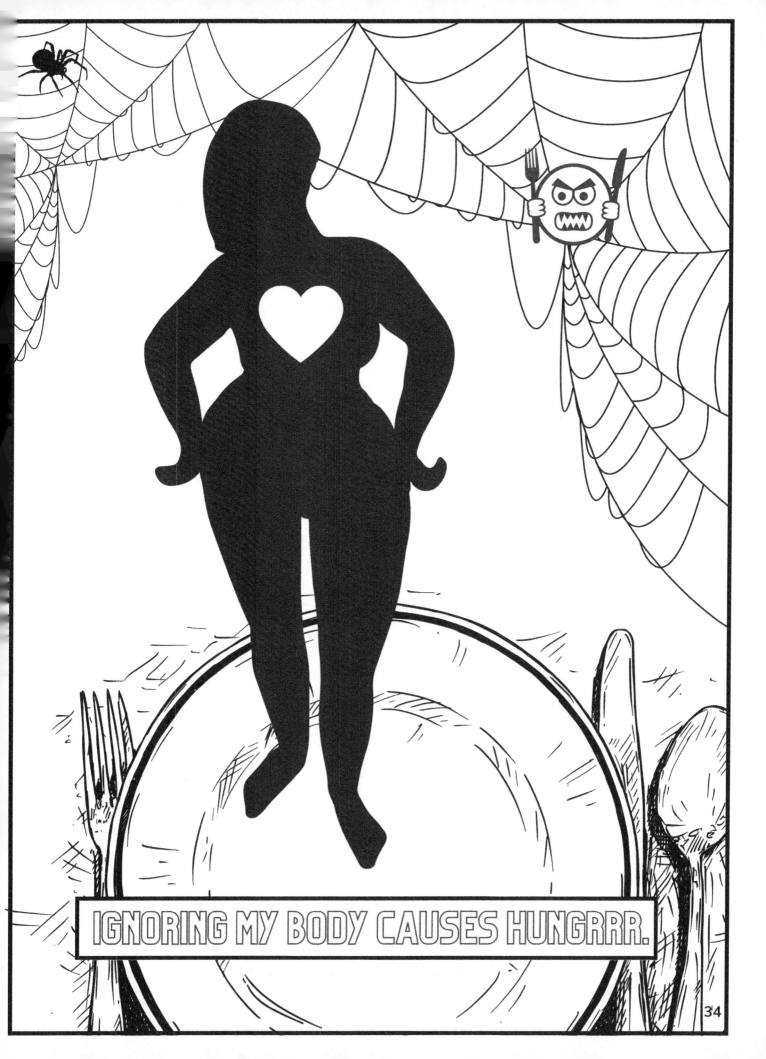

IGNORING MY BODY CAUSES HUNGRRR.

34

This Page Intentionally Left Blank

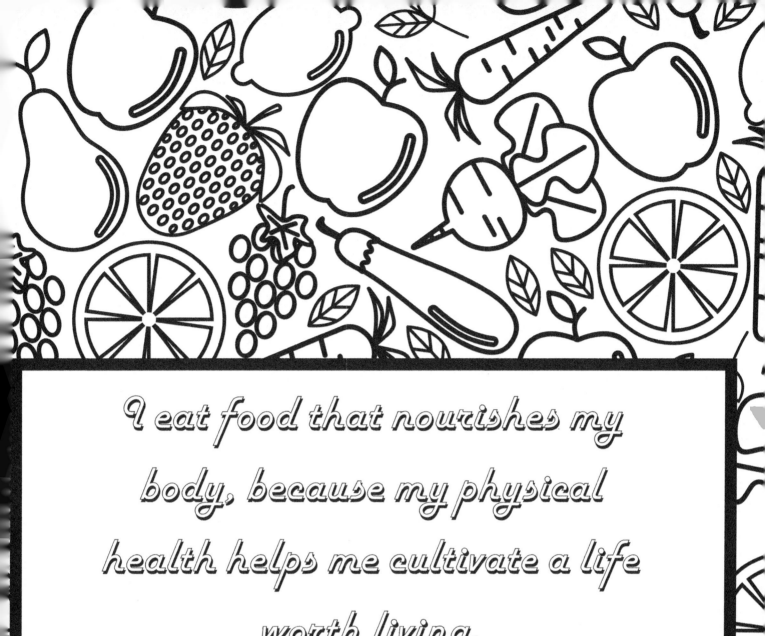

I eat food that nourishes my body, because my physical health helps me cultivate a life worth living.

37

How can my physical health support a life worth living?

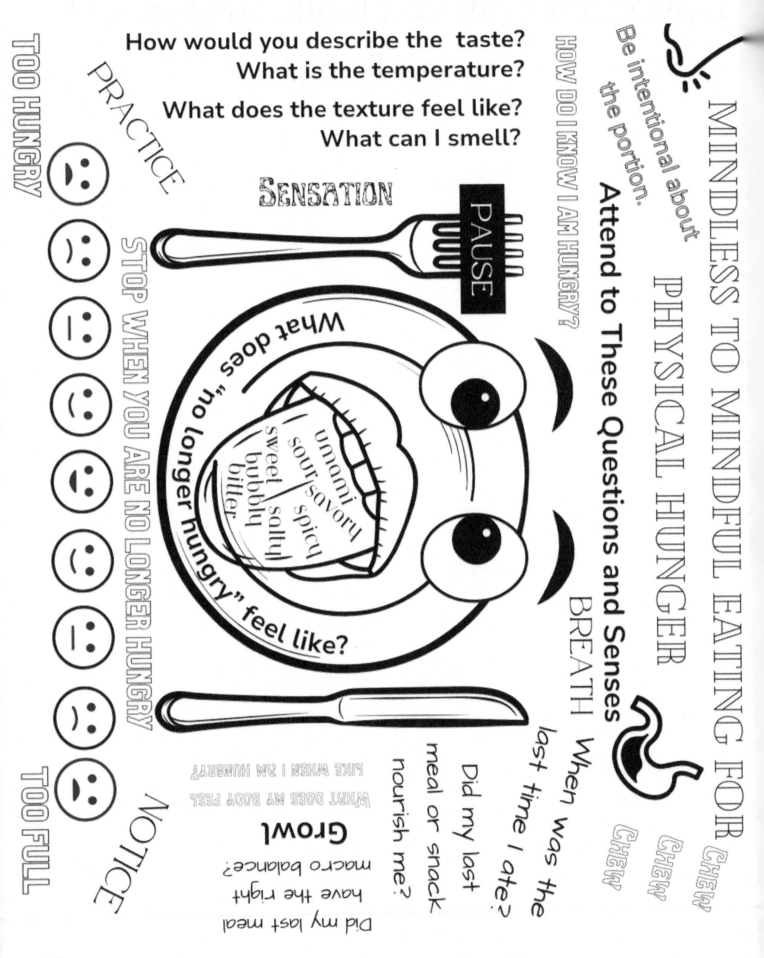

MINDLESS TO MINDFUL EATING FOR CHEW CHEW CHEW

PHYSICAL HUNGER

Be intentional about the portion.

Attend to These Questions and Senses

How would you describe the taste?
What is the temperature?
What does the texture feel like?
What can I smell?

SENSATION

PAUSE

HOW DO I KNOW I AM HUNGRY?

BREATH When was the last time I ate? Did my last meal or snack nourish me?

Growl
WHAT DOES MY BODY FEEL LIKE WHEN I AM HUNGRY?
Did my last meal have the right macro balance?

What does "no longer hungry" feel like?

umami
sour/savory
sweet spicy
bubbly salty
bitter

STOP WHEN YOU ARE NO LONGER HUNGRY

TOO HUNGRY

PRACTICE

NOTICE

TOO FULL

39

Mental Hunger

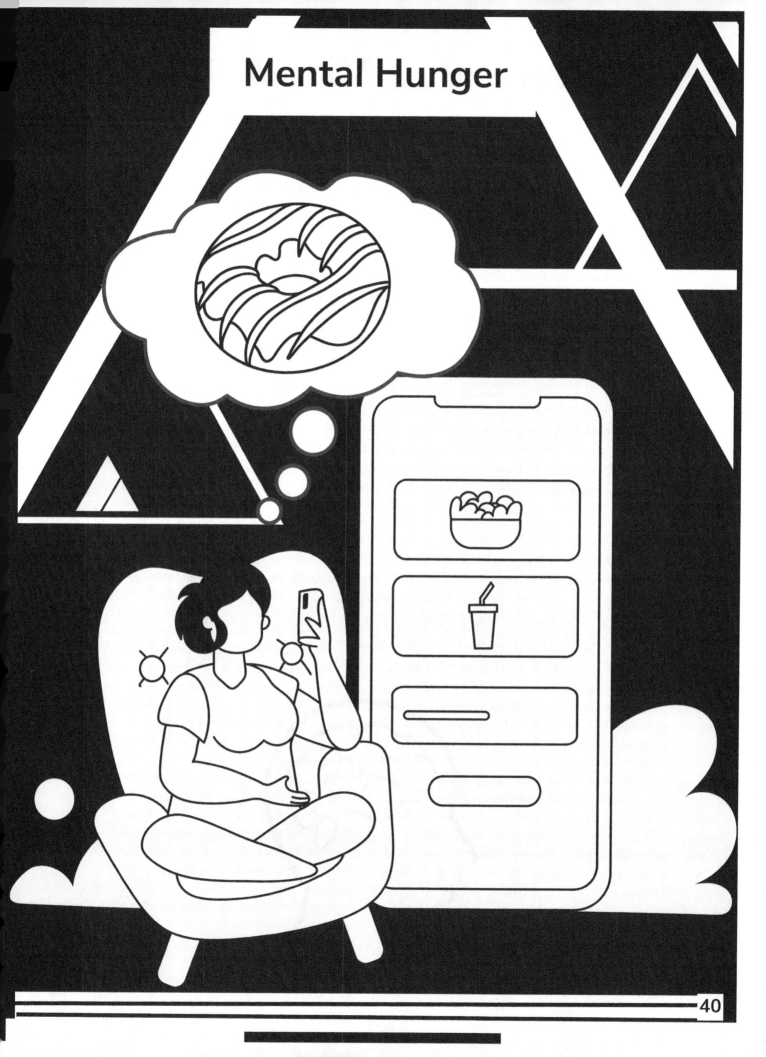

Understanding Mental Hunger

Mental hunger is a concept that describes our psychological desire to eat, even when our physical hunger is not present. It is the feeling of wanting to eat for reasons other than nourishment, such as boredom, stress, or cravings. Understanding mental hunger and its triggers can help us develop healthier eating habits and cultivate mindfulness in our daily lives.

One way to cultivate mindfulness is to be aware of our internal and external environments. Our internal environment includes our thoughts, emotions and physiological needs, while our external environment includes the people, places, and things around us. By being aware of these factors without judgment, we can better understand our eating behaviors and make more deliberate choices about what we eat.

For example, we may find ourselves reaching for candy and nuts on a road trip when we are tired. This is because chewing stimulates cognitive function and helps us stay awake. By recognizing this trigger, we can make a conscious decision to bring healthier snacks on our next trip or plan for rest stops to avoid mindless snacking.

External triggers are also common, such as seeing food in our environment and feeling the urge to eat it. This can happen when we walk through the kitchen and see a container of croissants on the counter or when we watch TV and see someone eating a hot fudge sundae. The novelty and perceived value of the item make us want it more, and this can lead to mindless eating.

The size of the dish can also impact how much we eat. Studies have shown that we tend to eat more when we are presented with larger portions, even if we are not physically hungry. This is because our brains perceive larger portions as more valuable and satisfying.

Cravings for specific flavors, such as salty, sweet, or spicy, or brand-named items can also be a result of habit. We may have developed a taste for these foods through previous experiences or marketing influences. By recognizing these patterns, we can make conscious choices to choose healthier alternatives or limit our intake of these foods.

In conclusion, cultivating mindfulness of our internal and external environments can help us make more deliberate choices about what we eat. By recognizing our triggers and being aware of our eating behaviors, we can develop healthier habits and improve our overall well-being.

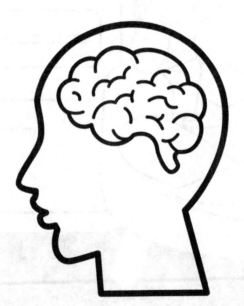

Can you recall an experience of mental hunger? Describe it.

This Page Intentionally Left Blank

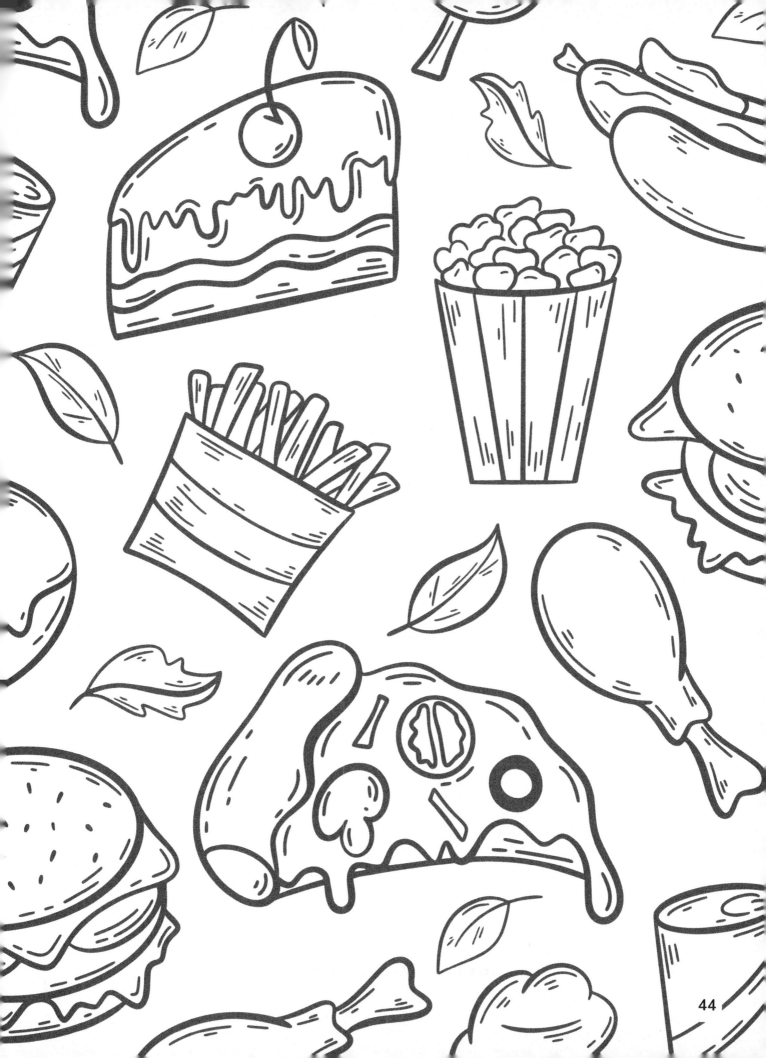

This Page Intentionally Left Blank

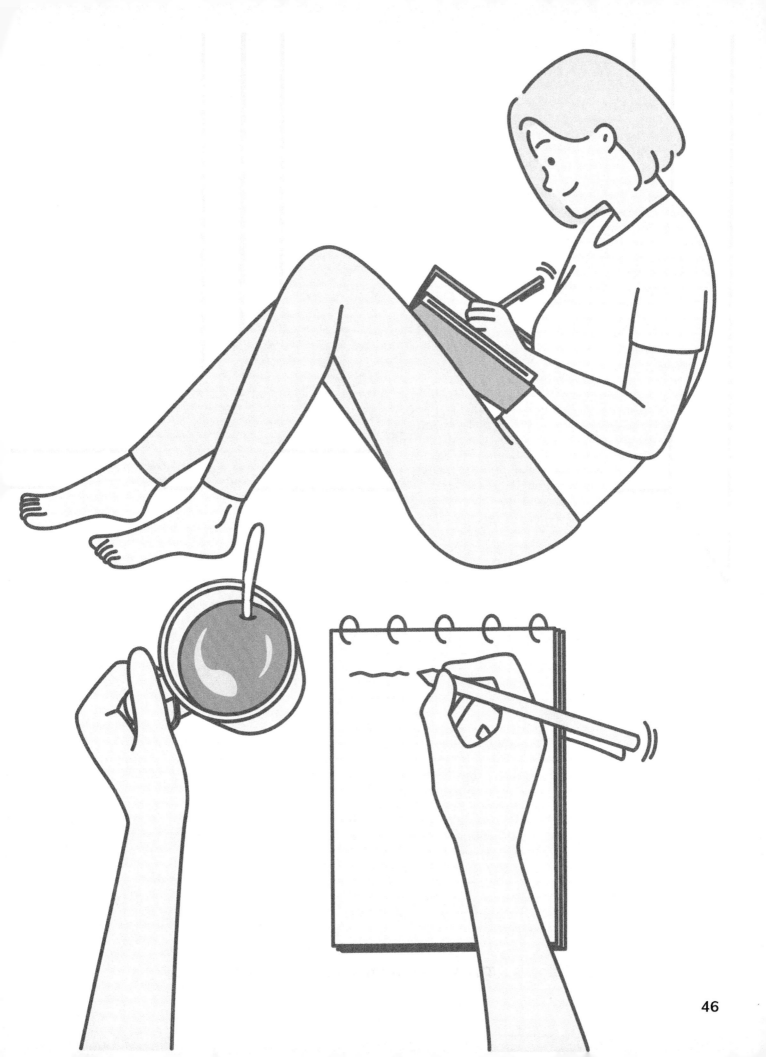

This Page Intentionally Left Blank

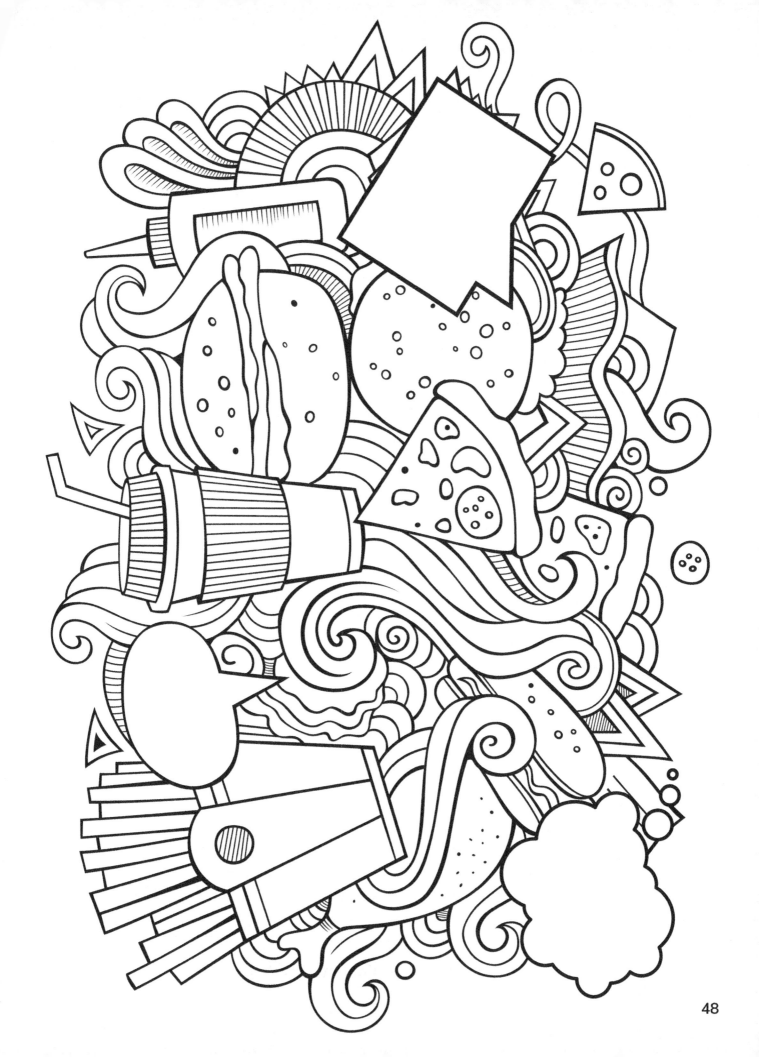

This Page Intentionally Left Blank

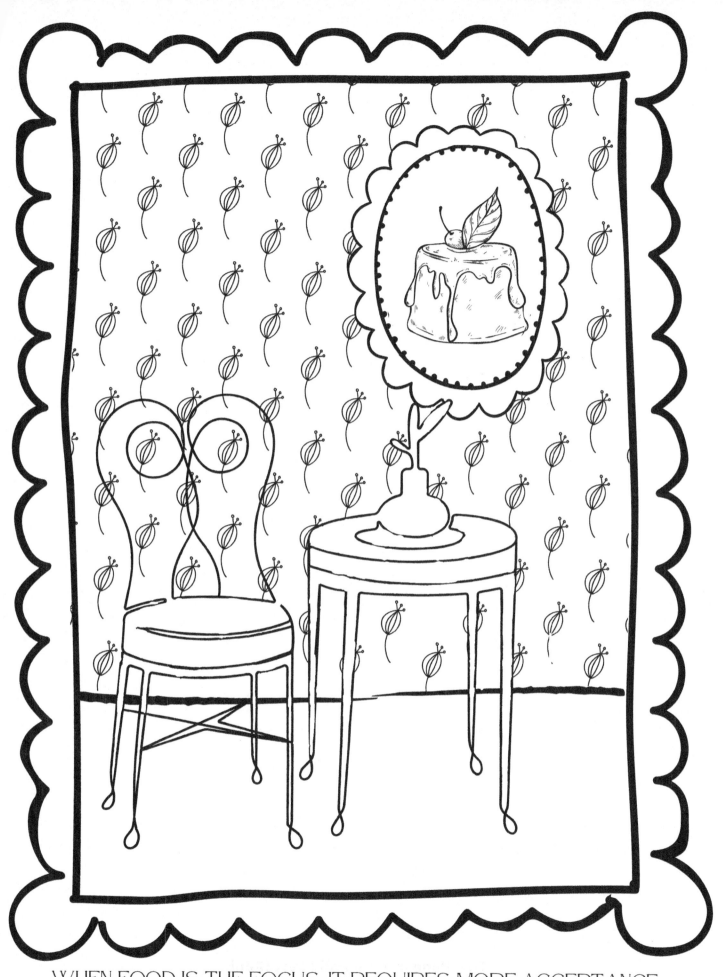

WHEN FOOD IS THE FOCUS, IT REQUIRES MORE ACCEPTANCE
AND INTENTIONALITY WITH CHOICES..

50

This Page Intentionally Left Blank

It is okay to savor the pleasure that food provides. When I impulsively stress eat, I stop savoring.

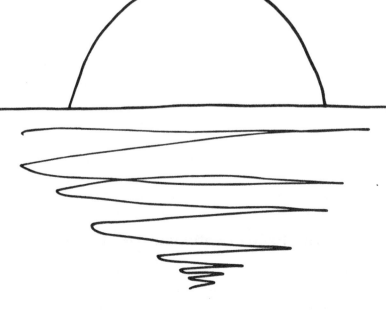

MINDLESS TO MINDFUL

I think I want...

FREE FOOD?!

EATING FOR MENTAL HUNGER

Where am I at?

SEE IT, WANNA EAT IT?

Attend to These Questions and Senses

DO I HAVE A TASTE FOR IT?

AM I EATING THIS JUST FOR FUN?

I hear someone cooking I hear something good

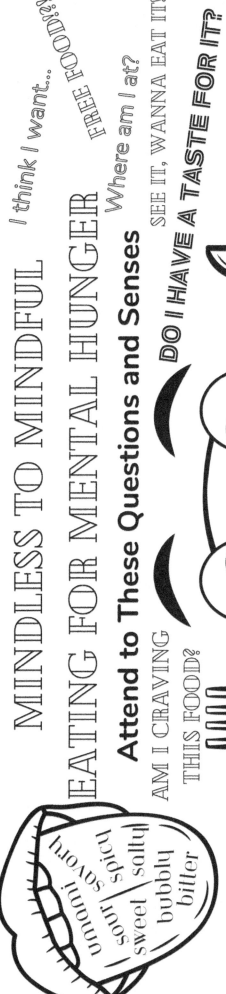

AM I CRAVING THIS FOOD?

Plate size

Size of the glass

What do other people think

Perceived abundance

NUMBER OF OPTIONS AVAILABLE

Portion Served

Value I place on it

WHAT'S THE MOUTH FEEL?

Who am I with?

Be intentional about the portion.

Did I see food on a screen recently?

AM I TRYING TO WAKE MYSELF UP?

umami
spicy
sour
sweet
salty
bubbly
bitter
savory

TIME OF DAY OR NIGHT

HOW MUCH WILL SATISFY ME?

AM I PHYSICALLY HUNGRY?

WHAT DO I THINK ABOUT IT?

How can I make this meal more intentional?

HOW MUCH DID THIS COST ME?

HOW MUCH DID SAVOR THE FLAVOR?

Am I on the dopamine roller coaster?

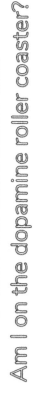

56

This Page Intentionally Left Blank

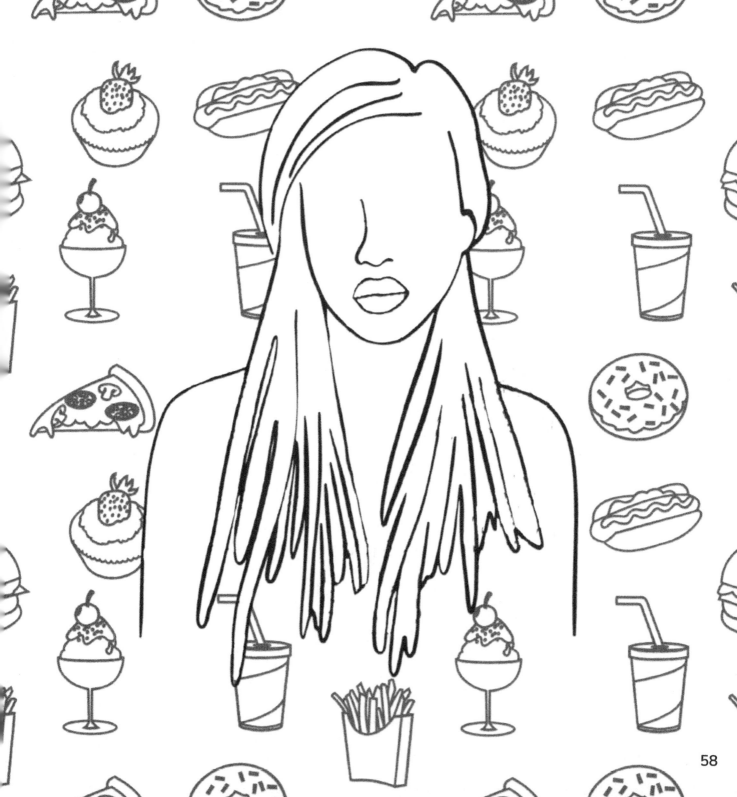

BE BRAVE
DEAR ONE. YOU WILL FIND
YOUR WAY OUT!

This Page Intentionally Left Blank

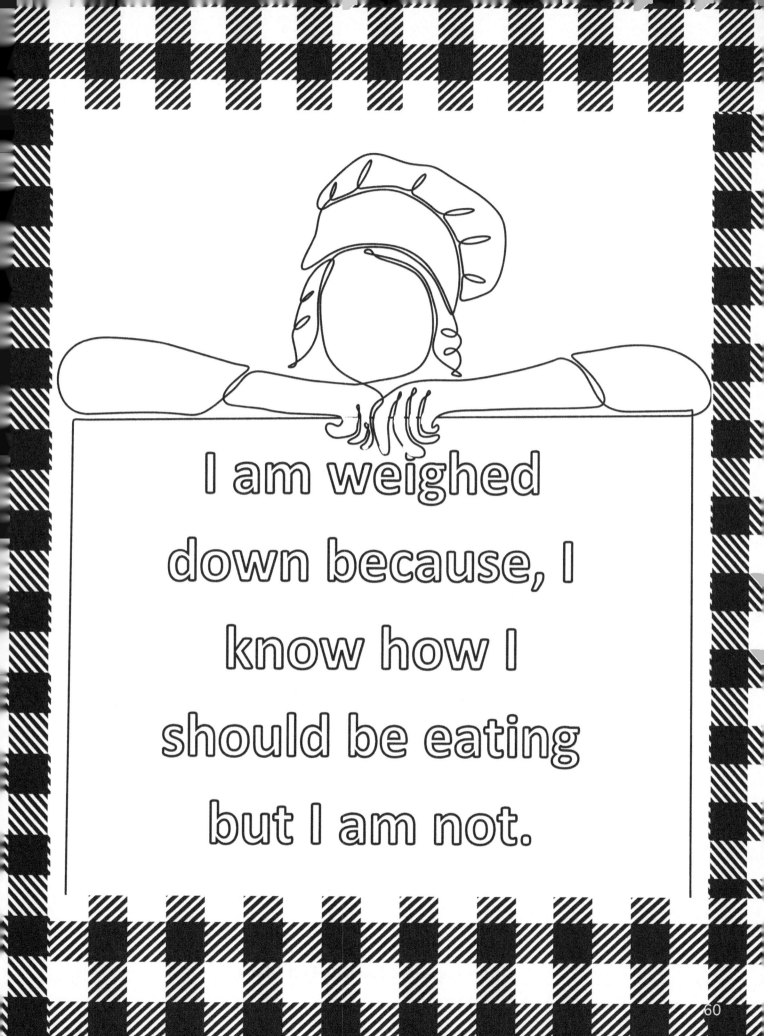

I am weighed down because, I know how I should be eating but I am not.

What foods am I eating in a way that I think I shouldn't?

What is that experience like for me? Physically, mentally and emotionally?

This Page Intentionally Left Blank

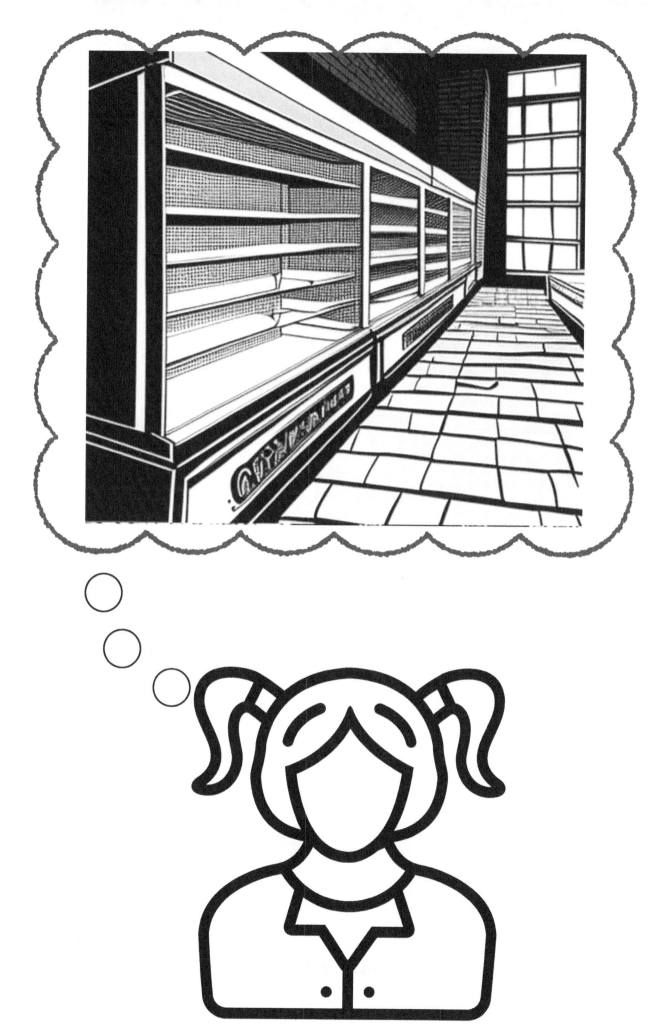

64

THERE IS AN ABUNDANCE OF NUTRITIOUS AND DELICIOUS FOOD AVAILABLE TO ME ANY TIME I WANT.

Have you ever experienced a scarcity of food? If so, how do you think it impacts your food choices now?

Emotional Hunger

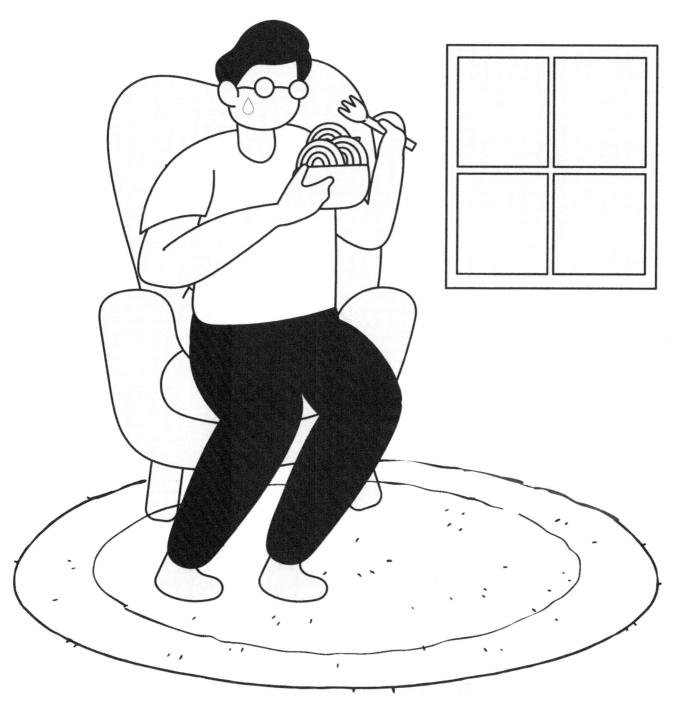

This Page Intentionally Left Blank

Understanding Emotional Eating
A Guide to Being Compassionate with Yourself

In our exploration thus far, we've discovered that relying on eating to regulate our energy and mood is a biological norm. However, it's crucial to recognize that this isn't always the ultimate solution for our mood or emotional well-being. Strategies that empower us to skillfully navigate and embrace our emotions, transforming them from potential adversaries into sources of strength are the skills we want to lean into when seeking to make changes in how, what and when we eat to regulate our mood and energy.

One aspect of emotional eating that merits deeper exploration is the pursuit of pleasure. Unfortunately, societal trends have distorted our understanding by labeling certain foods as "free," "skinny," or "zero calorie," creating an altered reality where we pretend to experience the pleasure of a meal without truly feeling it. When we stigmatize certain foods as forbidden or bad, we inadvertently link eating that food to a moral or behavioral failing. All too often that results in some unkind self talk. And this is where things need to stop! Rather than hurting yourself, you need to support yourself.

In reality, once we've experienced the pleasure of foods like ice cream or warm baked bread with butter, our brains remember that joy.

Enhancing our relationship with ourselves, our environment, and our health involves the ability to say both YES and NO to pleasurable foods. This means embracing the reality of cravings and then confidently saying YES or NO, and trusting that we can eat the craved food in a healthful way or the craving will pass. Remember, cravings are suggestions, not commandments. The decision to say YES or NO is personal and depends on various factors.

During discussions about emotional eating, emotions like grief, shame, and fear often surface. As humans, we all grapple with painful emotions that sometimes feel overwhelming. Drawing inspiration from Rumi, who proclaimed, "the wound is the place where the light enters you," we can view significant wounds as opportunities for profound growth and transformation.

In the realm of emotional eating, two primary factors drive the behavior: seeking to reduce uncomfortable feelings or intensifying positive ones. Understanding these motives is crucial in untangling the complex web of emotions entwined with our relationship with food.

The journey involves learning to feel our emotions without judgment and cultivating a compassionate attitude toward ourselves. This transformative process encourages a deeper understanding of the self, fostering emotional resilience and paving the way for healthier coping mechanisms. Embracing our emotions becomes a powerful tool in navigating the intricate landscape of emotional eating with greater self-awareness and compassion.

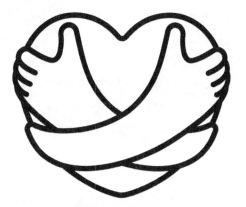

Intimately Acquainted with Stress
Unveiling the Facts and Resources

Stress is a familiar companion that weighs upon us and leaves its mark on our lives. The mere mention of its negative impact on our health can even amplify our existing stress levels. However, my purpose is to equip you with factual knowledge and valuable resources to bolster your ability to manage stress effectively.

It is evident that when we lack adequate stress management tools or resort to harmful coping mechanisms, the repercussions on our overall well-being are significant. Particularly, when food becomes our primary refuge, it can shift from a source of solace to an unhealthy dependency. This dependency is not just behaviorally driven, it is influenced by the workings of our biology and how it interacts with the chemistry of food.

During moments of stress, our inclination is often to seek out foods rich in sugar, starch, and fat, which, produces high levels of serotonin and dopamine. These neurotransmitters improve our mood in the moment, yet, when the sugar, starch, and fat is consumed excessively, can harm our bodies. This perpetuates a distressing cycle that fosters a sense of entrapment and hopelessness. Personally, I have experienced this struggle, and as a nutritionist, I have witnessed countless individuals feeling powerless in the face of their emotions and their connection with food. To break free from this cycle, we must intervene early in the cycle, identifying the emotional triggers and embracing the desire to change the cycle. Below, you will find a simplified illustration of this cycle. By intervening at the emotional trigger and our desire to feel something different, we hold the power to reshape the outcome and pave the way for positive transformation.

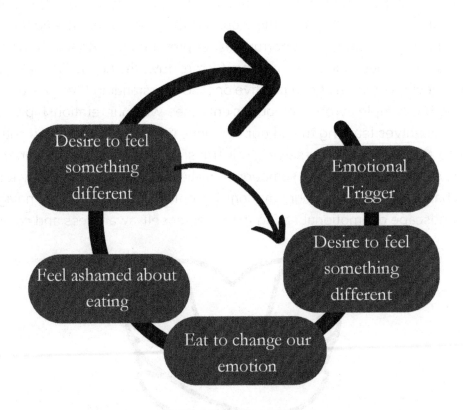

Mastering Emotional Coping
Effective Strategies for Surfing the Urge of Stress Eating

To navigate the intricate landscape of emotions and effectively manage stress eating, we can embrace an array of coping strategies derived from renowned therapeutic modalities like Dialectical Behavioral Therapy (DBT) and Cognitive Behavioral Therapy (CBT). These evidence-based approaches provide valuable tools for understanding and managing our emotional well-being. By integrating the principles and techniques of DBT and CBT into our lives, we can cultivate greater emotional resilience, self-awareness, and overall psychological wellness. Drawing from my experience in providing nutrition counseling for nearly a decade, I have found the following techniques to be particularly effective in helping you surf the urge of stress eating:

Dialectical Behavioral Therapy (DBT) skills: DBT offers valuable tools for anxiety regulation, such as those outlined in resources like Intrepid Mental Health's blog or in a DBT therapy group near you. These skills include:

- Radical Acceptance: Embrace things as they are, recognizing that change can only happen when we acknowledge reality.
- Willingness: Approach necessary actions without resisting or expending excessive energy in opposition.
- Participate One Mindfully: Engage fully in the present moment, free from the burdens of the past or concerns about the future.
- Minimize susceptibility to emotional eating episodes with the help of the **PLEASE** acronym, incorporating these essential practices into your routine:
  - **Prioritize Physical Health**: Pay attention to your overall well-being by taking care of your physical health. This involves nurturing your body through activities that promote physical vitality.
  - **Address Illnesses**: Be proactive in addressing any underlying illnesses or health concerns. Seek appropriate medical attention, follow prescribed treatments, and ensure you are taking necessary steps to manage any conditions effectively.
  - **Embrace a Balanced Diet**: Nurture your body with a balanced and nourishing diet. Focus on consuming a variety of wholesome foods that provide the necessary nutrients for optimal physical and mental functioning. Maintain a healthy relationship with food by practicing mindful eating and being attuned to your body's hunger and fullness cues.
  - **Steer Clear of Mood-Altering Substances** (this includes certain foods): Be mindful of the impact substances like alcohol, drugs, or excessive caffeine can have on your emotional well-being.
  - **Cultivate Quality Sleep and Exercise**: Prioritize quality sleep to support your body's recovery and rejuvenation. Establish consistent sleep routines and create a conducive sleep environment. Additionally, incorporate regular exercise into your lifestyle, as it helps reduce stress, boost mood, and enhances overall well-being.

Harnessing the Power of Cognitive Behavioral Therapy (CBT) and Overcoming Cognitive Distortions

CBT enlightens us on the profound influence our thoughts and beliefs wield over our emotions. Recognizing and addressing cognitive distortions, which impede personal growth, empowers us to identify and confront unconstructive thinking patterns.

Throughout my experience in nutrition counseling, I have frequently encountered several prevalent cognitive distortions:

1. All-or-nothing thinking: This cognitive distortion manifests as a tendency to view situations in extremes, perceiving outcomes as either entirely positive or entirely negative, without room for nuance or gray areas.

2. Perfectionism: Individuals afflicted by perfectionism strive for flawlessness, setting unrealistically high standards for themselves. Any perceived imperfections or shortcomings are often magnified, leading to self-criticism and diminished self-esteem.

3. The Tyranny of Shoulds: This distortion involves placing excessive emphasis on rigid expectations and demands, both from oneself and others. This can create an unrelenting pressure to conform to arbitrary standards, causing distress and a sense of failure when unable to meet these expectations.

4. Self-criticism: Individuals struggling with self-criticism have a propensity for harshly judging themselves, focusing on perceived faults and inadequacies. This negative self-talk can contribute to feelings of unworthiness and undermine self-confidence.

By recognizing these cognitive distortions and understanding their impact on our thoughts, emotions, and behaviors, we can challenge their validity and replace them with more balanced and constructive thinking patterns. Through intentional effort and therapeutic techniques, we can cultivate healthier perspectives, bolster self-compassion, and foster personal growth.

Embarking on this transformative journey through the pages of this coloring book, our aim is not to shame or suppress our desires for food, nor to deny the psychological pleasure it brings. Instead, we empower ourselves to make conscious choices. Rather than viewing a container of ice cream as an item to be strictly avoided, fearing that indulgence will lead to self-judgment and disappointment for not exercising restraint, we embrace the ice cream as a source of pleasure, then we recognize the power within us to confidently say NO or YES and lean into other non food coping tools.

At the core, our approach centers on complete acceptance of food as an intrinsic part of our lives. We consciously craft the unfolding story of our relationship with food, embracing its role while honoring our own preferences and well-being. This journey encourages us to find balance, cultivate mindfulness, and foster a harmonious connection with the nourishment that sustains us. With each stroke of color, let us celebrate the complexities and joys of our culinary experiences, savoring the transformative power that lies within our conscious choices.

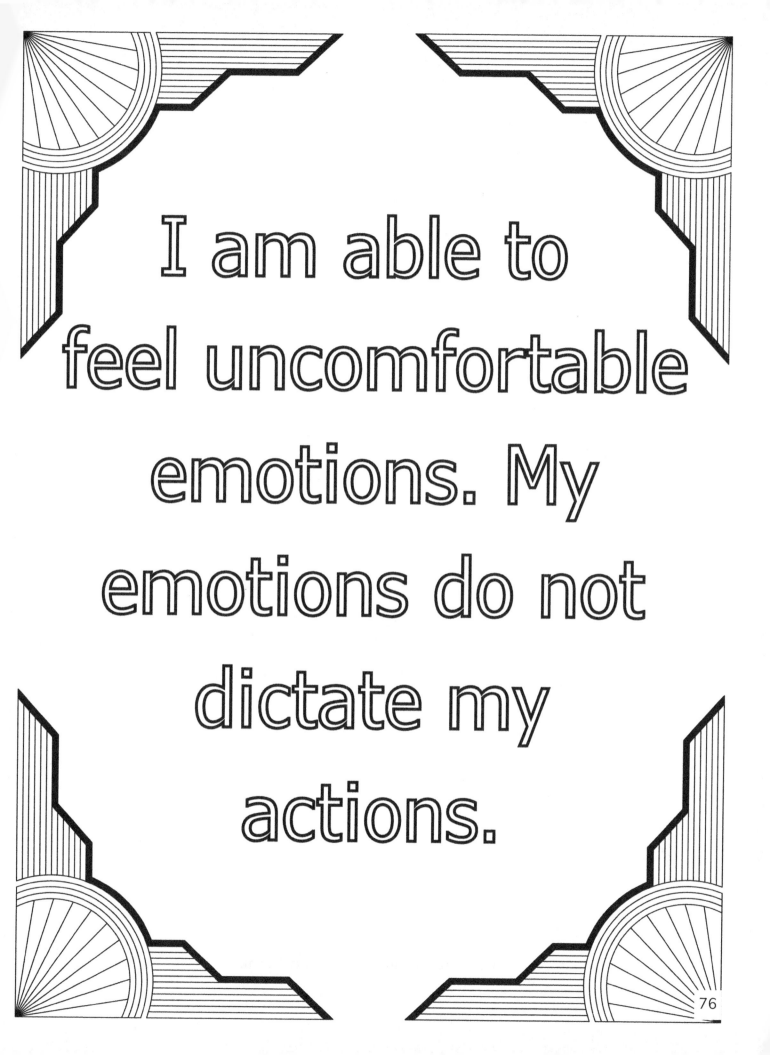

I am able to feel uncomfortable emotions. My emotions do not dictate my actions.

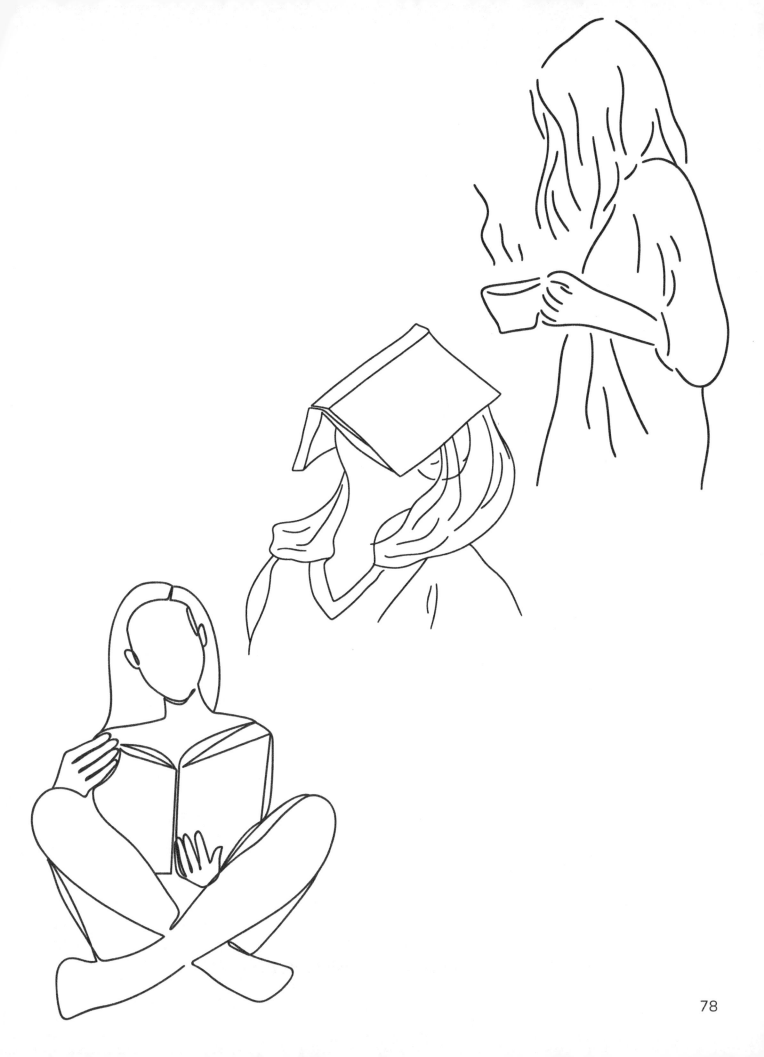

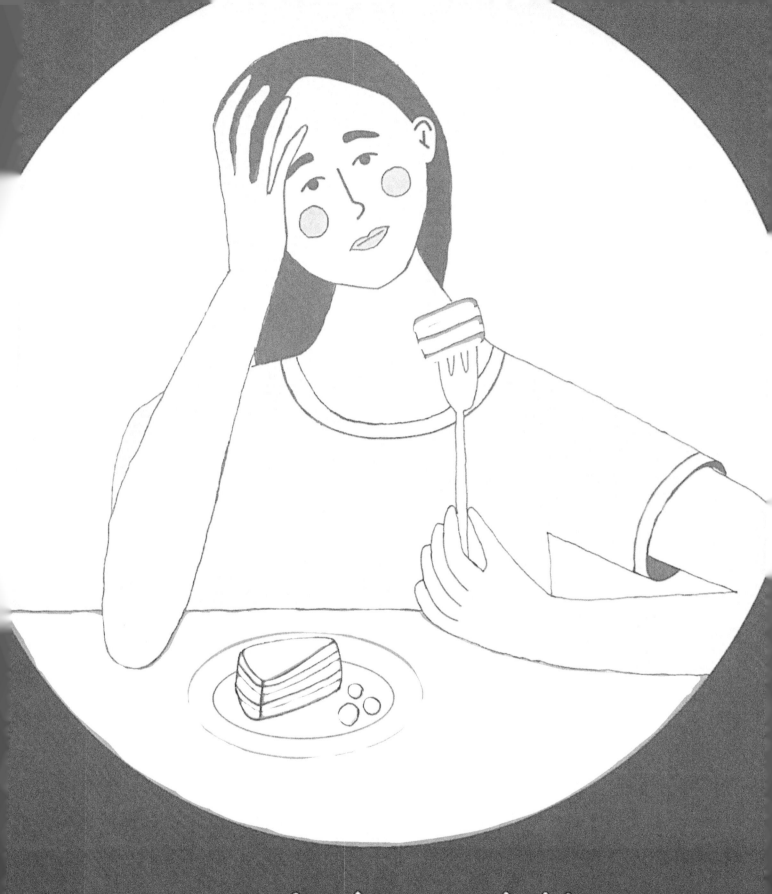

I really wish it wasn't this way...

This Page Intentionally Left Blank

Is there something you are having a hard time accepting? Remember, with acceptance the struggle ceases and opportunity opens up.

This Page Intentionally Left Blank

Never Say Never to growth.

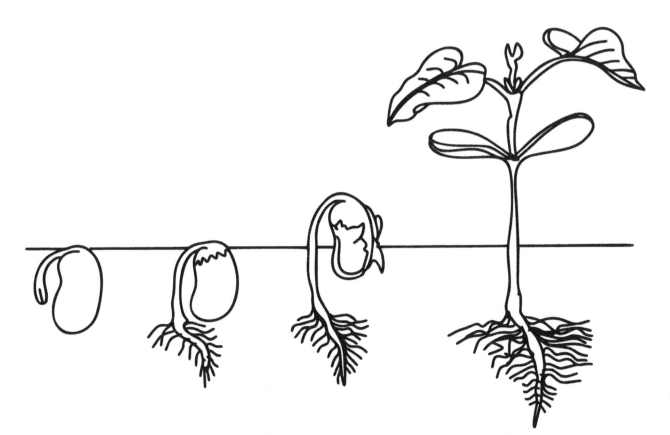

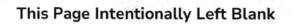

This Page Intentionally Left Blank

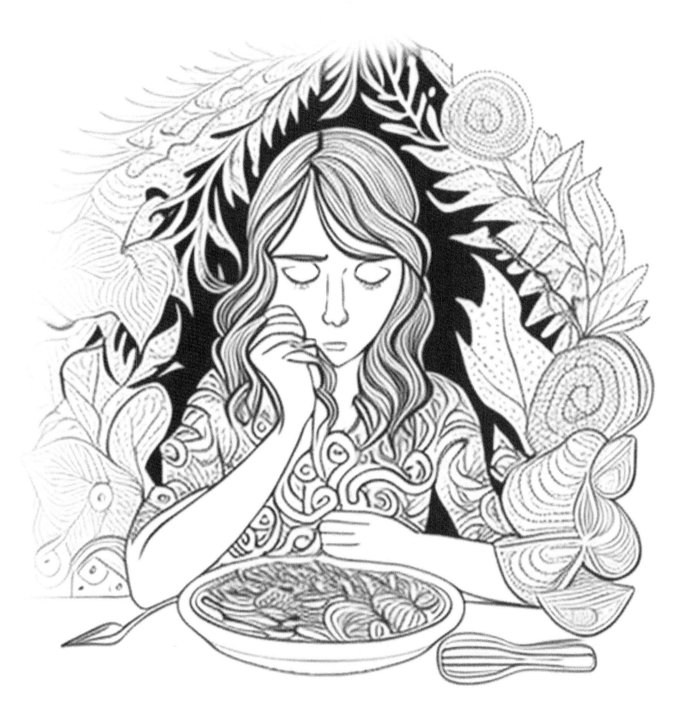

I WISH I FELT HUNGRY, I WISH I KNEW WHAT TO EAT, WHY I AM ALWAYS IN THE DARK.

This Page Intentionally Left Blank

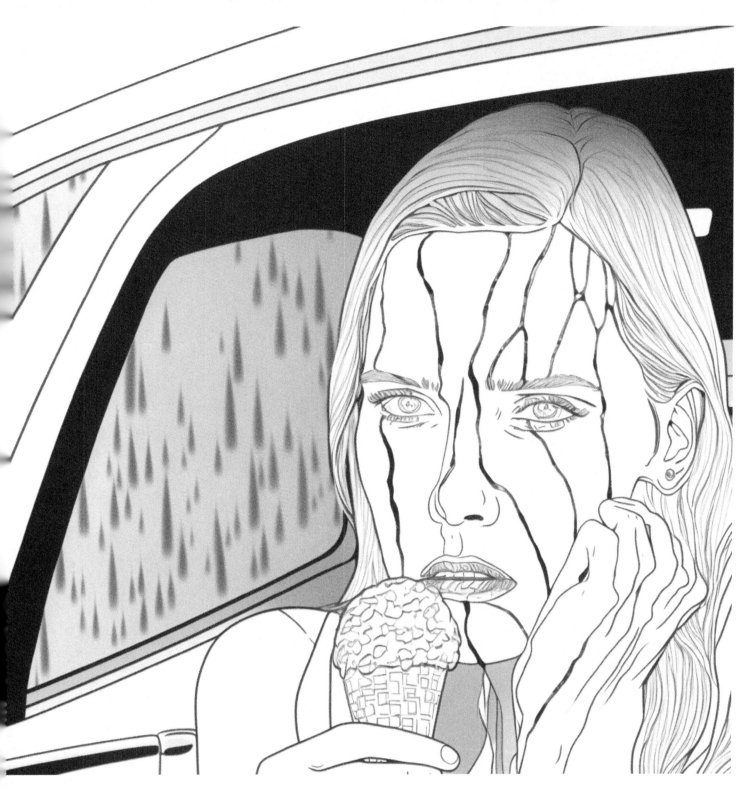

Am I just spinning my wheels? I keep doing this, I really do want to change. I am ready to do this differently.

This Page Intentionally Left Blank

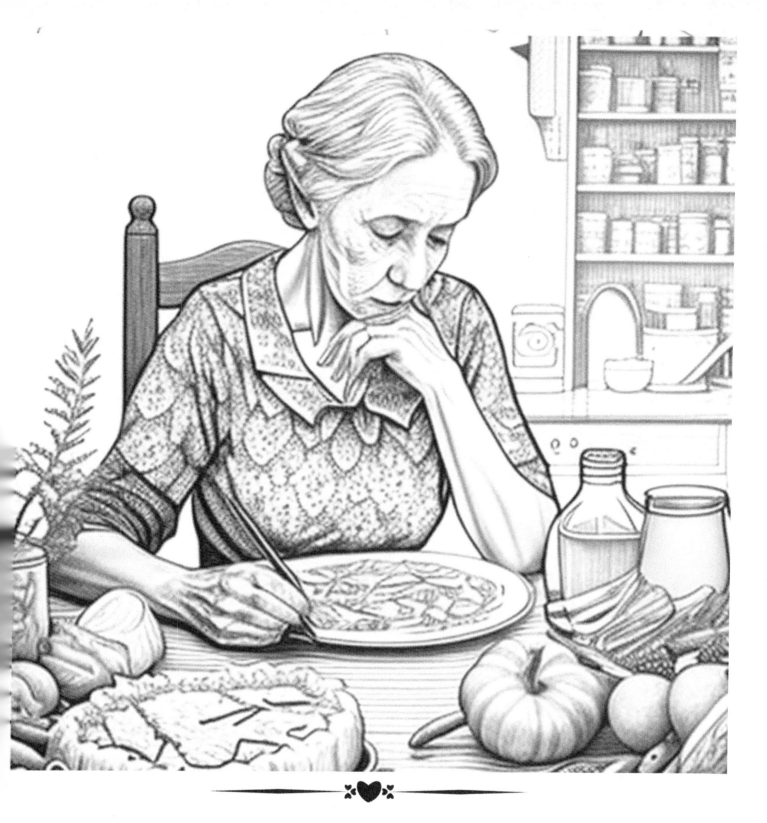

It is never too late or the wrong time to examine your relationship with self nourishment or your relationship with food.

This Page Intentionally Left Blank

Mindful Eating for Emotional Hunger

Am I trying to feel a certain emotion?

AM I TRYING TO RESTORE MY DEPLETED ENERGY?

WHAT AM I LOOKING TO GET OUT OF THIS MEAL?

CAN I SLOW DOWN?

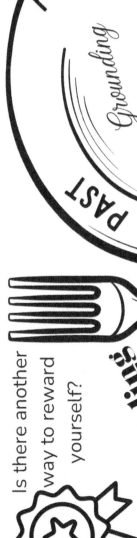

FUTURE

Grounding

WHERE AM I?

Healing

Connecting

PAST

PRESENT

Feeling is Healing

RIDE THE CRAVE WAVE

Am I punishing yourself with this food choice?

Stop and Smell the Rose Tea!

Is it food that I really need?

Where in my body do I feel this hunger?

Is there another way to reward yourself?

Avoid Avoiding

Am I Restricting? Binging? Grazing?

A Craving is Just an Urge

Is there a feeling driving this hunger?

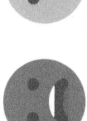

Is this an empowering or disempowering choice?

This Page Intentionally Left Blank

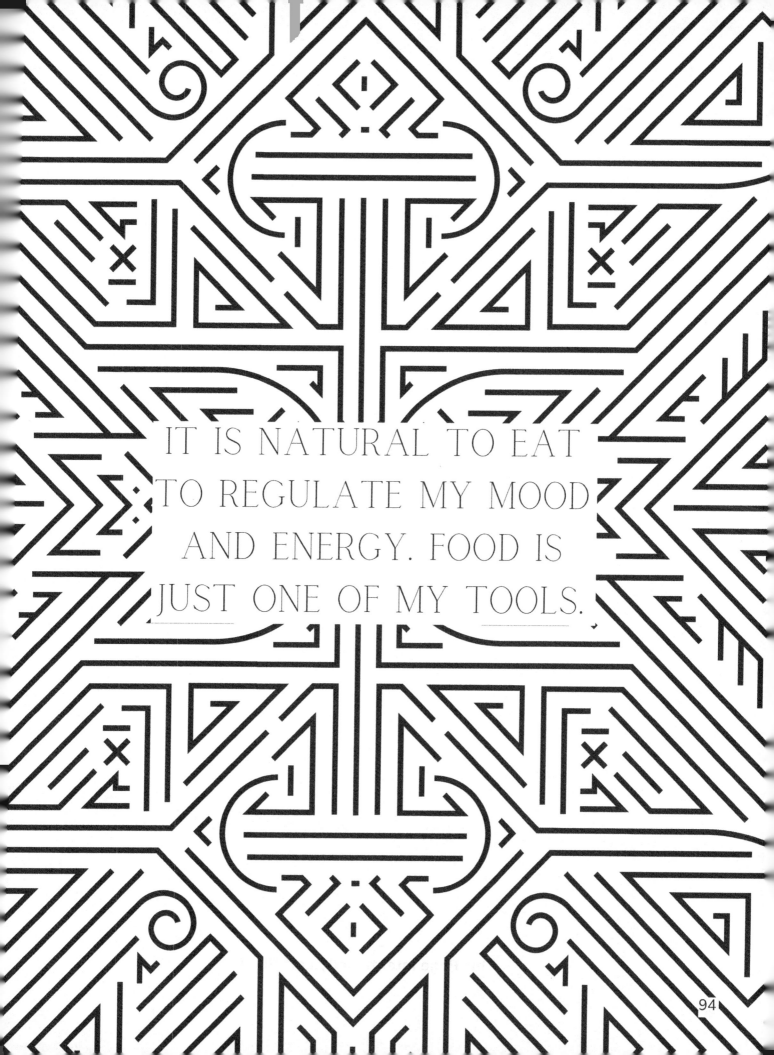

IT IS NATURAL TO EAT
TO REGULATE MY MOOD
AND ENERGY. FOOD IS
JUST ONE OF MY TOOLS.

This Page Intentionally Left Blank

My Personal Hunger Cues
Mental

Emotional

Physical

Part III

Surfing the Urge

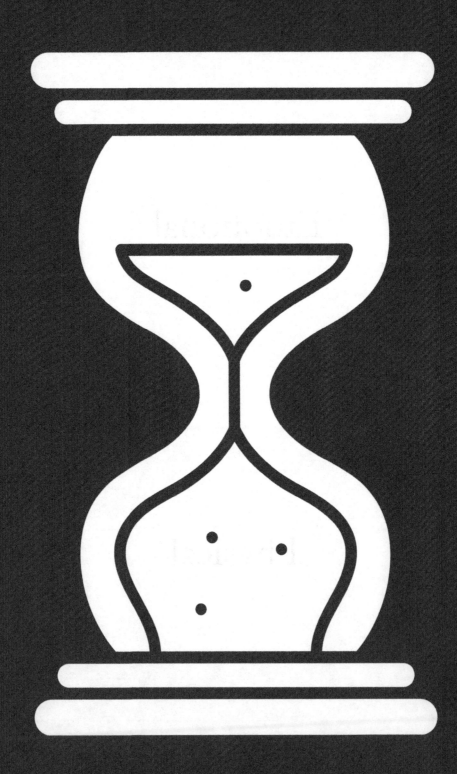

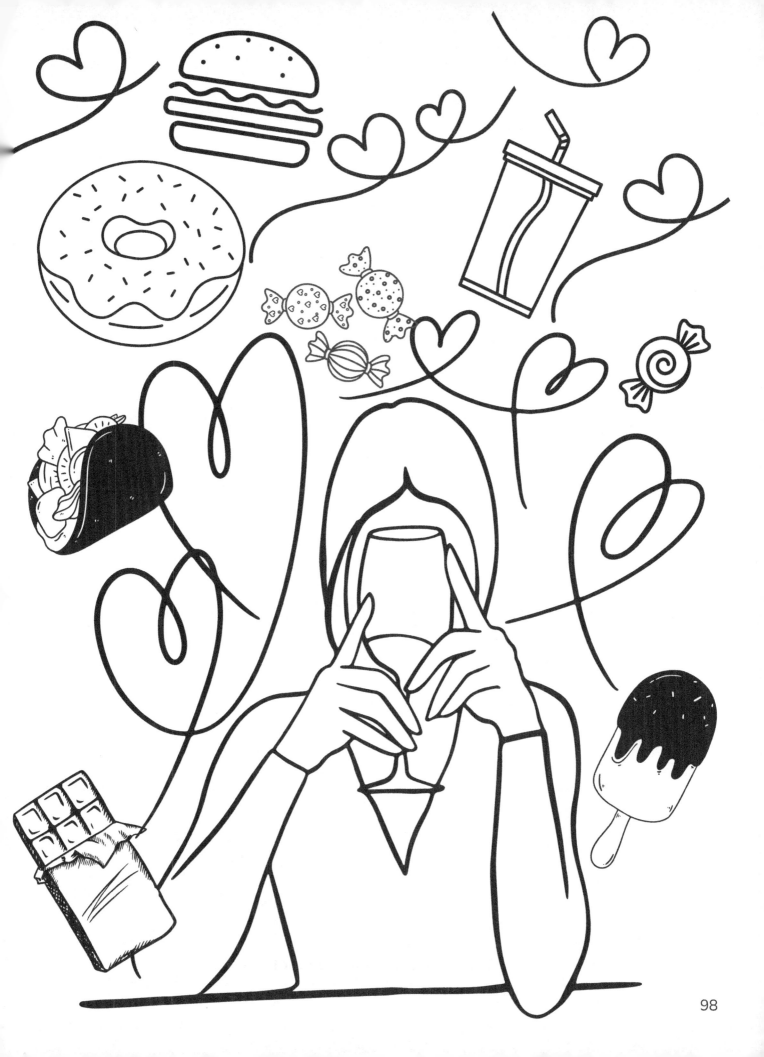

This Page Intentionally Left Blank

I am a part of the whole universe. I have the inner strength to choose a path. I am willing to commit to that path. I can do things differently.

Deal With Cravings Using the 6 D's

Shine a light on food cravings with this simple 6 step strategy to deal with food cravings.

1. Determine-Question the facts, do you really need the food or is it a want?

2. Describe to yourself what the experience was the last time you ate this food. What was the outcome?

3. Delay-Set a timer and see if you are still having the craving in 20 minutes.

4. Distract-If you've decided that you want to avoid eating, then concentrate on something else.

5. Distance-Create space between yourself and the tempting food.

6. Decide-If you are going to eat, choose to eat in a way that is in alignment with your health goals, such as how much to eat, then enjoy it.

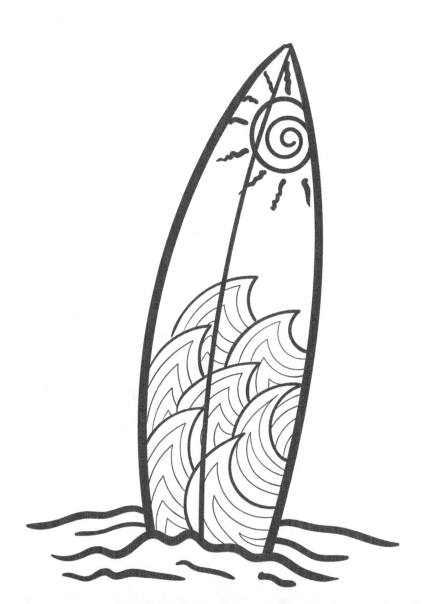

Practice Presence

With a mindful countdown: 5,4,3,2,1

In moments when we find ourselves emotionally overwhelmed, consumed by repetitive thoughts, and burdened with stress, it's important to explore alternative ways to ground and center ourselves. One powerful mindfulness practice that can be utilized anytime and anywhere is the sensory grounding exercise. This exercise engages our senses and redirects our attention to the present moment, allowing us to regain clarity and find inner calm.

Here's an example of how to practice the sensory grounding exercise: Take a moment to pause and bring your awareness to your surroundings.

- Begin by identifying and focusing on five things you can see around you. It could be objects in your immediate environment, nature outside, or people nearby. Pay attention to their colors, shapes, and textures.
- Next, shift your attention to four things you can touch. It might be the texture of your clothing, the sensation of a surface beneath your fingertips, or the warmth of a cup in your hand. Notice how each object feels against your skin.
- Then, bring your awareness to three things you can hear. Listen carefully to the sounds in your environment, whether it's the gentle hum of the air conditioner, distant traffic, or the rustling of leaves. Take in each sound without judgment.
- Move on to two things you can smell. Focus on any scents present in your surroundings, such as the aroma of coffee, fresh flowers, or the scent of the outdoors. Breathe in deeply and notice the specific qualities of each smell.
- Finally, concentrate on one thing you can taste. It could be the lingering flavor in your mouth from a recent meal, a piece of gum, or even just the natural taste of your breath. Pay attention to the sensations on your tongue as you focus on this taste.

By engaging your senses through this mindfulness exercise, you can anchor yourself in the present moment, redirect your focus away from distressing thoughts, and cultivate a sense of calm and presence.

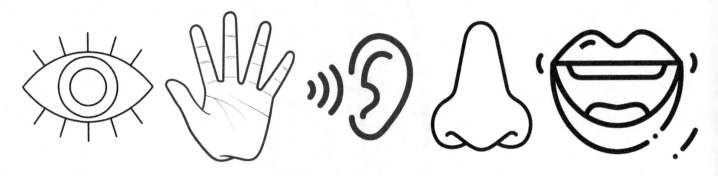

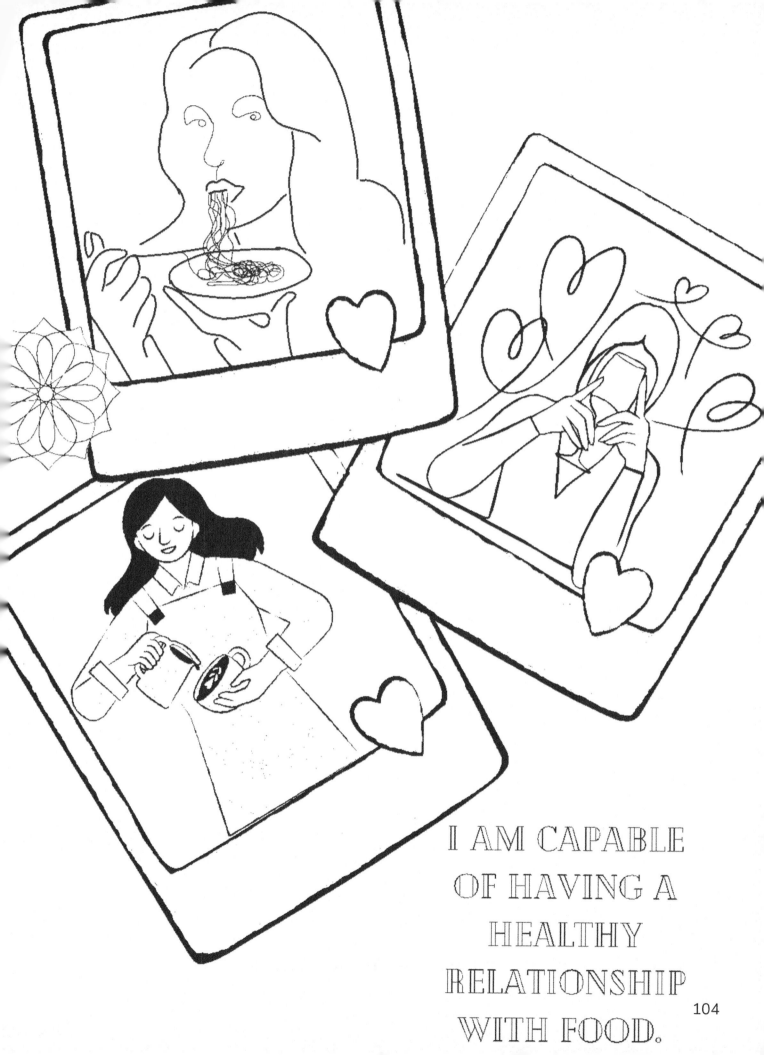

I AM CAPABLE OF HAVING A HEALTHY RELATIONSHIP WITH FOOD.

104

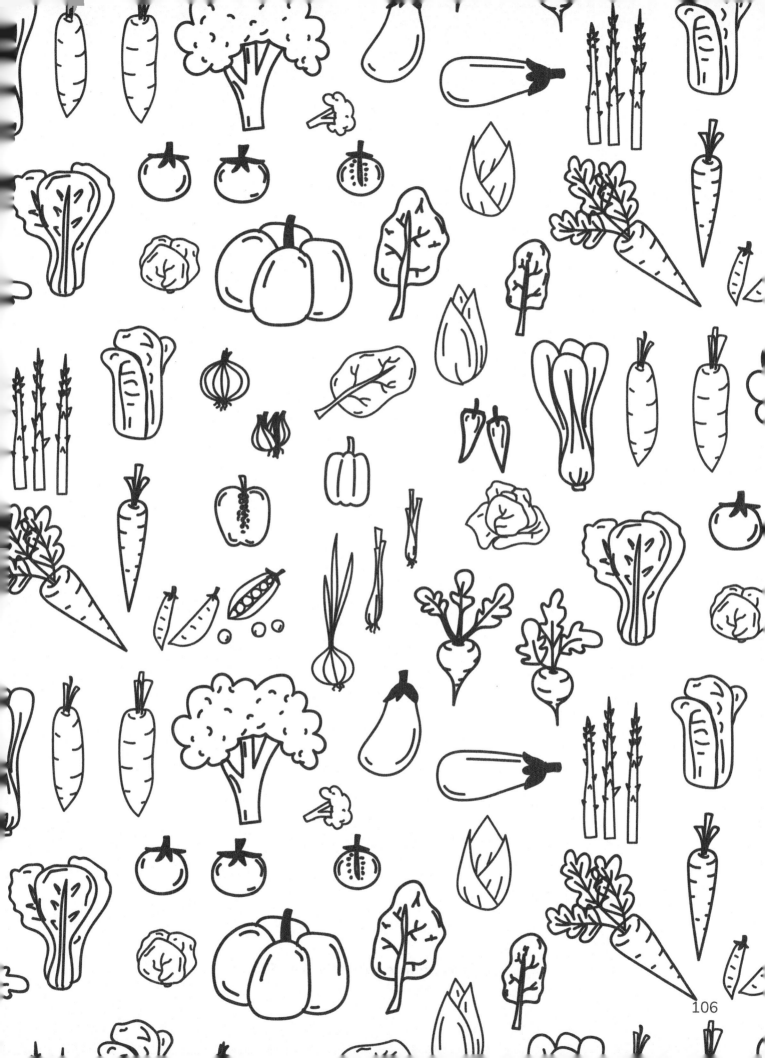

This Page Intentionally Left Blank

EAT WHAT YOU WANT, ADD WHAT YOU NEED.

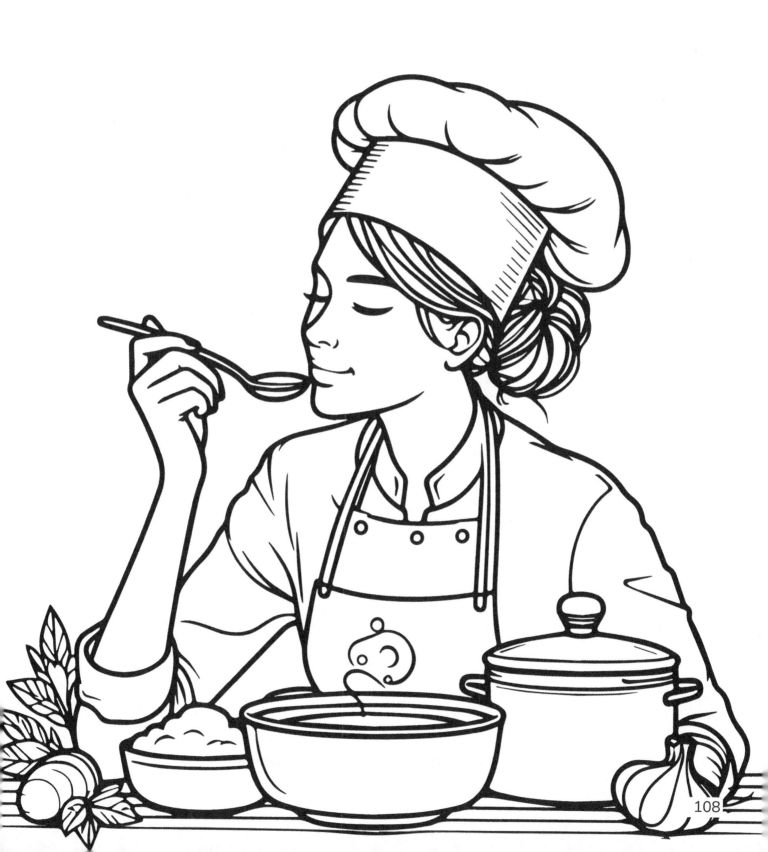

This Page Intentionally Left Blank

Non-Food Based Strategies

We need to develop non-food based hobbies, loves, rewards, distractions and soothies in order to truly surf the urge. Here is a list to get started with, please feel free to add to it.

1. Color a page in this book, then post it proudly to social media.
2. Create a piece of collage art.
3. Learn a new skill such as "how to draw your favorite animal".
4. Knit a granny square.
5. Go shopping.
6. Play a video game.
7. Text someone, something kind and supportive.
8. Call a friend and ask about their day.
9. Go for a walk with a friend.
10. Do yoga or some other type of stretching.
11. Breath.
12. Stand outside and feel the wind blow away any unwanted thoughts/feelings.
13. Listen to music.
14. Pray.
15. Focus on the belief, I am not alone and ask for what you need to make it through this situation.
16. Meditate on a candle flame.
17. Practice mindfully engaging in an activity, like vacuuming or driving.
18. Day dream, imagine something pleasant.
19. Imagine a time when your body felt healthy.
20. Do some journaling about the emotions you are feeling.
21. Reflect on the purpose or value in this stressful situation.
22. Take a hot bath or shower.
23. Snuggle up in your favorite pajamas, get into bed, pull the covers over your head and cry.
24. Make a cup of hot herbal tea and mindfully sip it.
25. Take a break from pain, focus on something pleasurable.
26. Be your own best friend and give yourself a pep talk, what is it you need to hear?
27. Grab your favorite essential oil and mindfully breath it in.
28. Give yourself a foot rub.
29. Go buy yourself flowers.
30. Look at cute cat pictures.
31.
32.
33.
34.
35.
36.
37.

My Self Care Kit

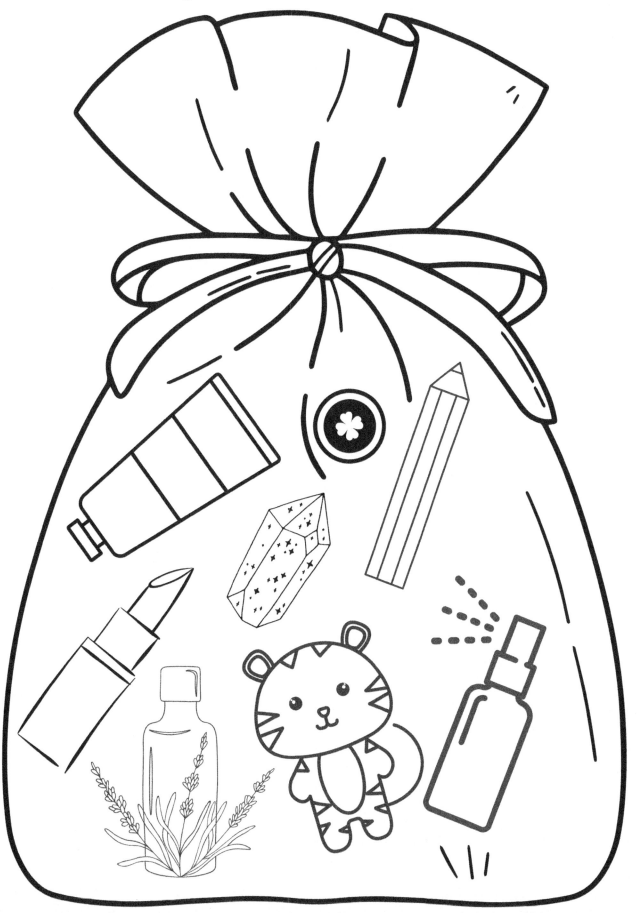

My Plan:

When Stress Strikes

I will use one or all of these 4 non-food items soothe me?

_____

_____

_____

_____

I also have these 4 activities can I do besides eat?

_____

_____

_____

_____

If I need to consume something to de-escalate feeling overwhelmed, what 4 foods/beverages are reasonable, allowed and part of a healthy plan?

_____

_____

_____

_____

I have these 5 senses can I tune into to regain my presence?

_____

_____

_____

_____

This Page Intentionally Left Blank

In a perfect world, what does a healthy relationship with food feel like to you?

What behaviors or thoughts would help you feel that way? Be as specific as possible.

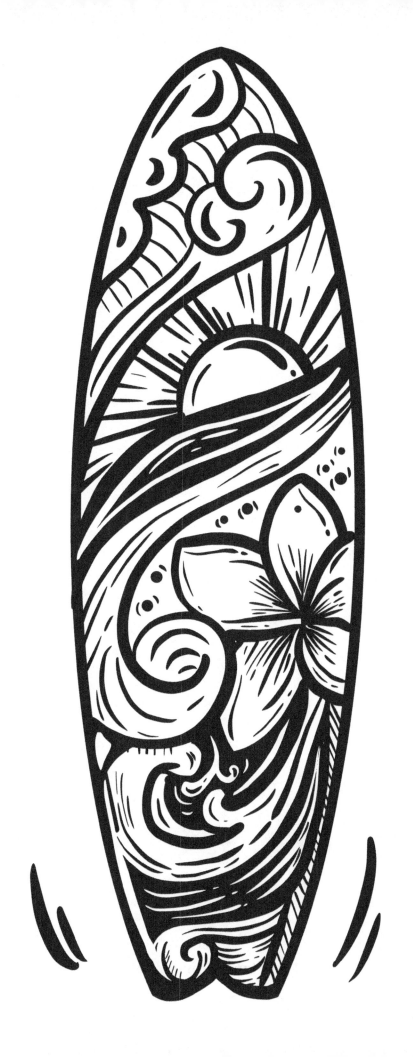

This Page Intentionally Left Blank

I am able to eat and drink in a way that fulfills my mental, emotional and physical being.

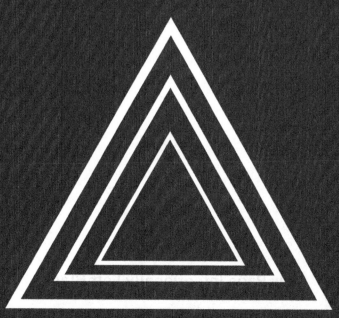

This Page Intentionally Left Blank

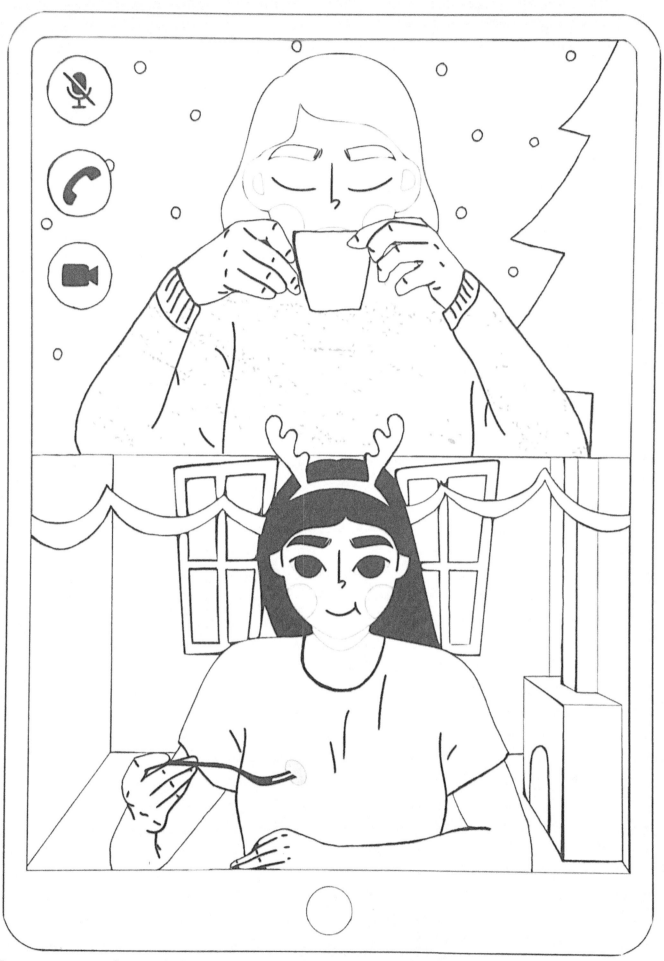

I am comfortable with my food story in social situations.

What are you getting from eating or drinking the food items you crave?

"It is impossible to understand addiction without asking what relief the addict finds, or hopes to find, in the drug or the addictive behaviour."
-Dr. Gabor Mate

This Page Intentionally Left Blank

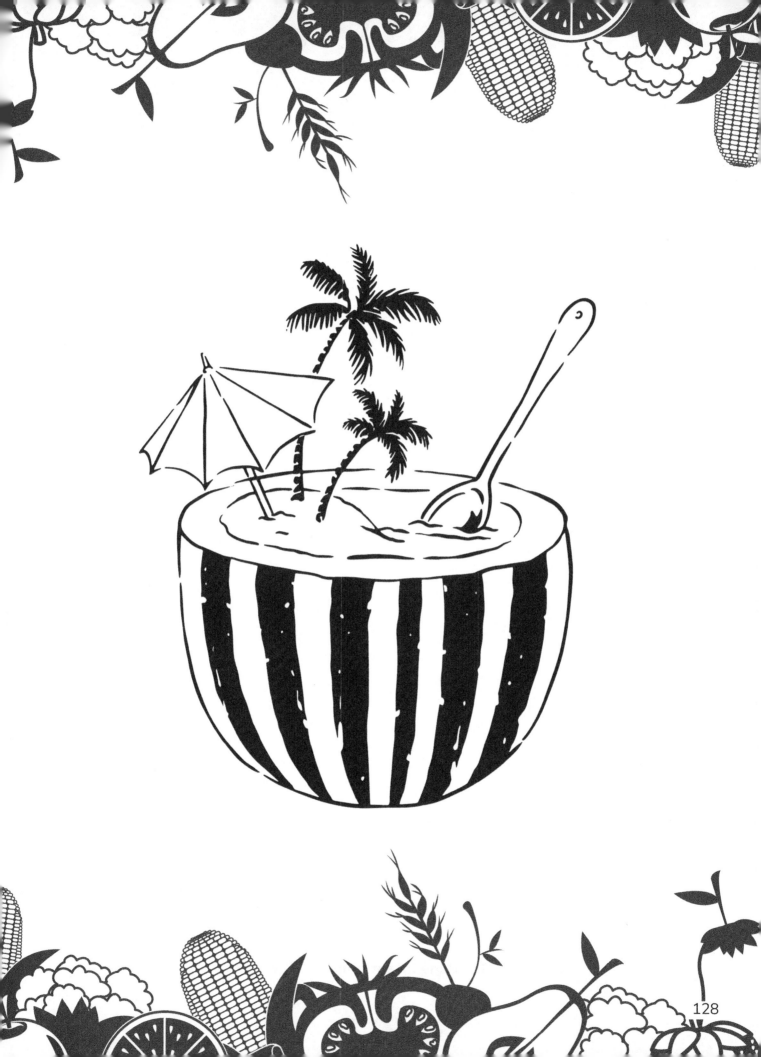

Is there something I am avoiding or resisting feeling?

This Page Intentionally Left Blank

"You can't stop the waves but you can learn to surf."

— John Kabat-Zin

133

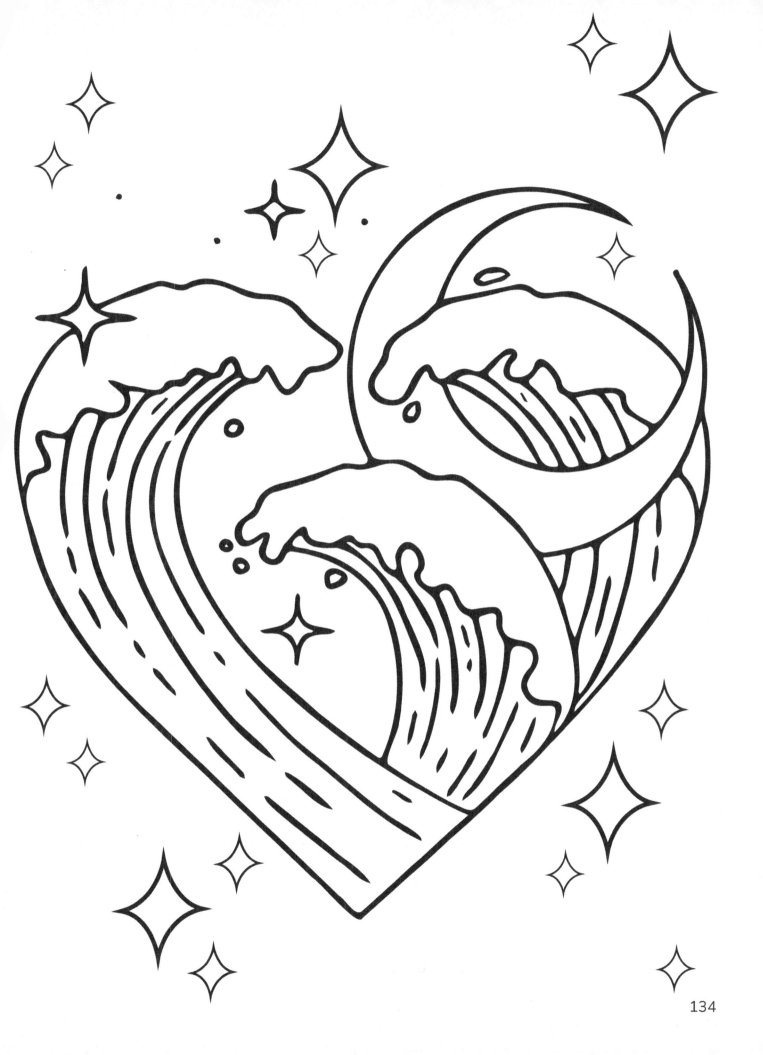

This Page Intentionally Left Blank

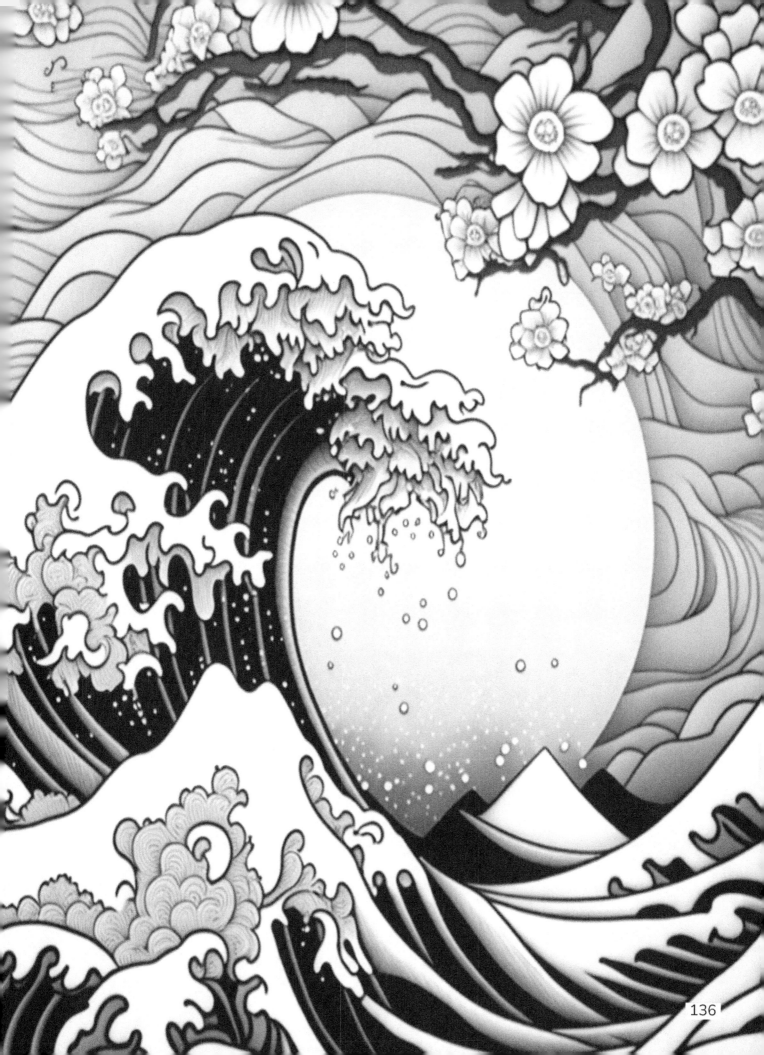

This Page Intentionally Left Blank

What you resist, persists. -Carl Jung

This Page Intentionally Left Blank

I am willing to:

This Page Intentionally Left Blank

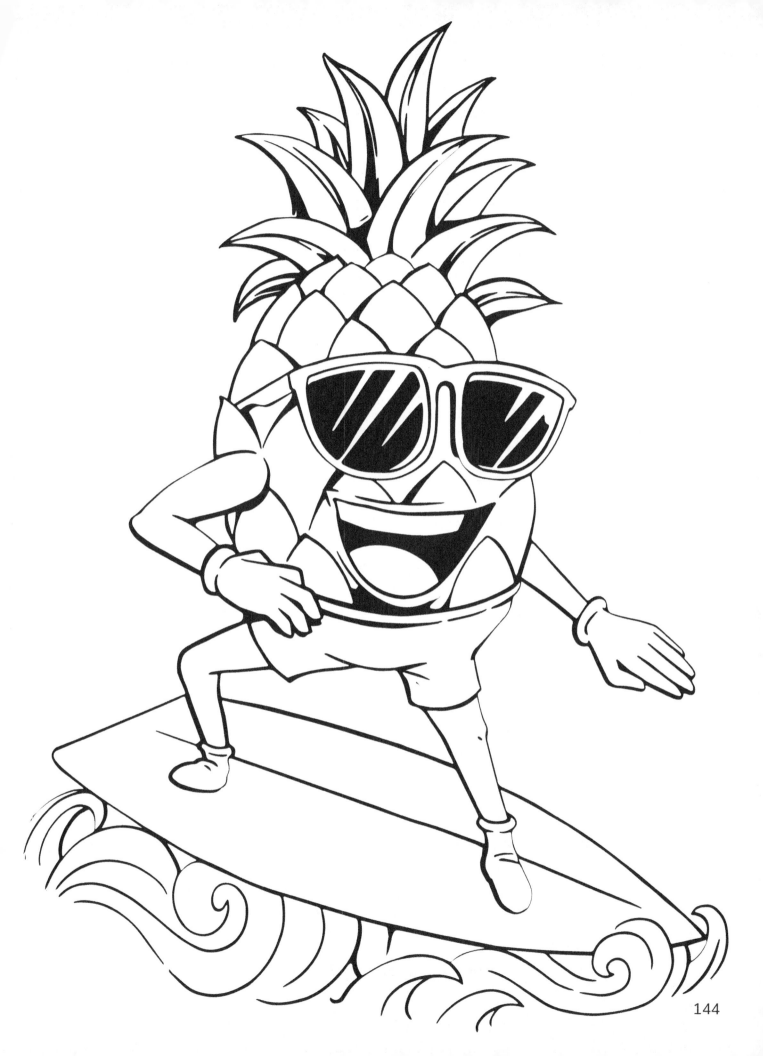

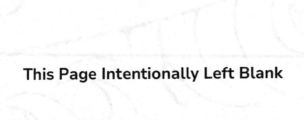

This Page Intentionally Left Blank

Ways I am beginning to stay mindful and present:

This Page Intentionally Left Blank

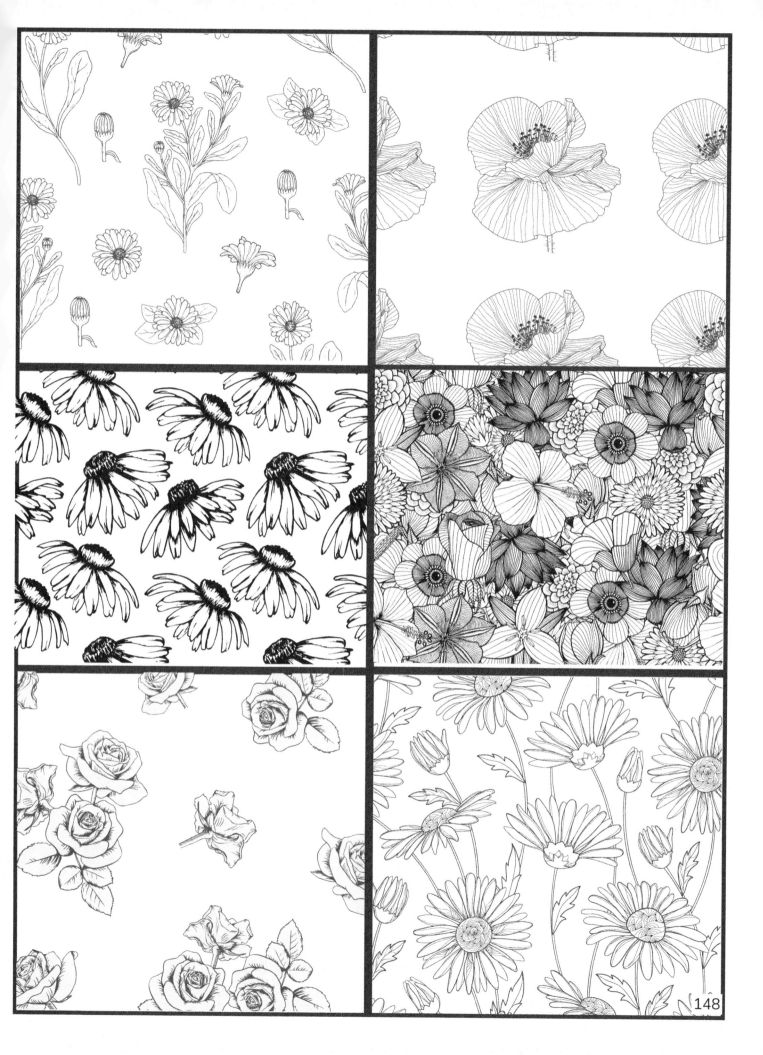

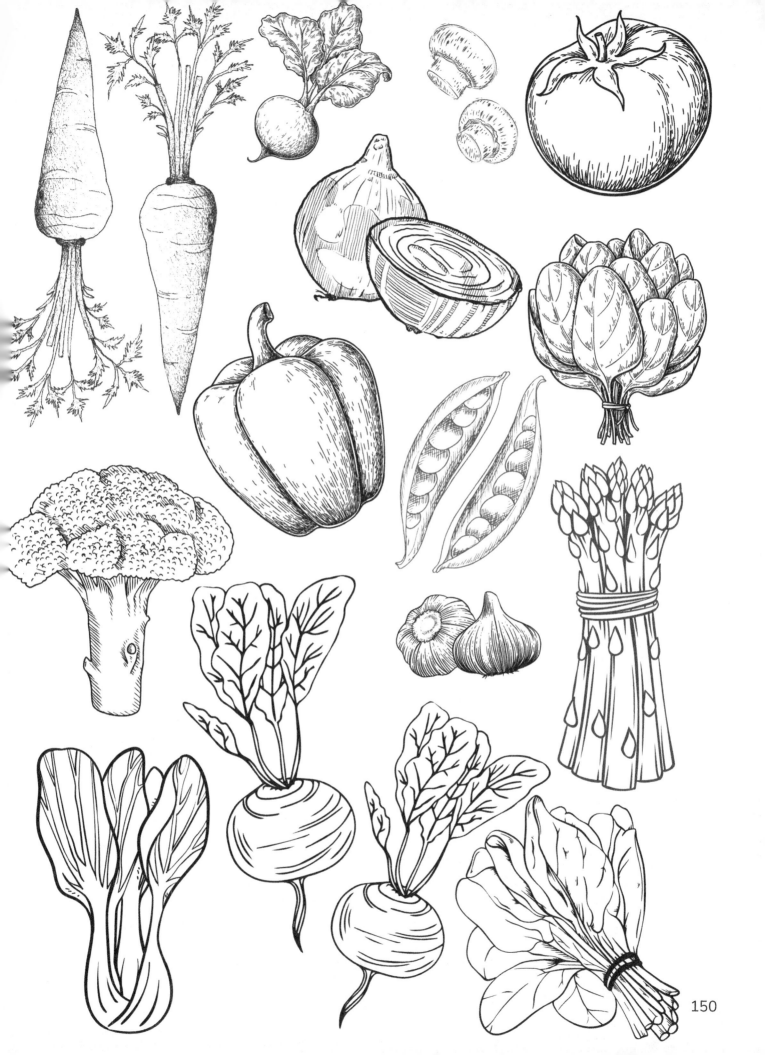

This Page Intentionally Left Blank

Part IV
Reclaiming the
Sacred

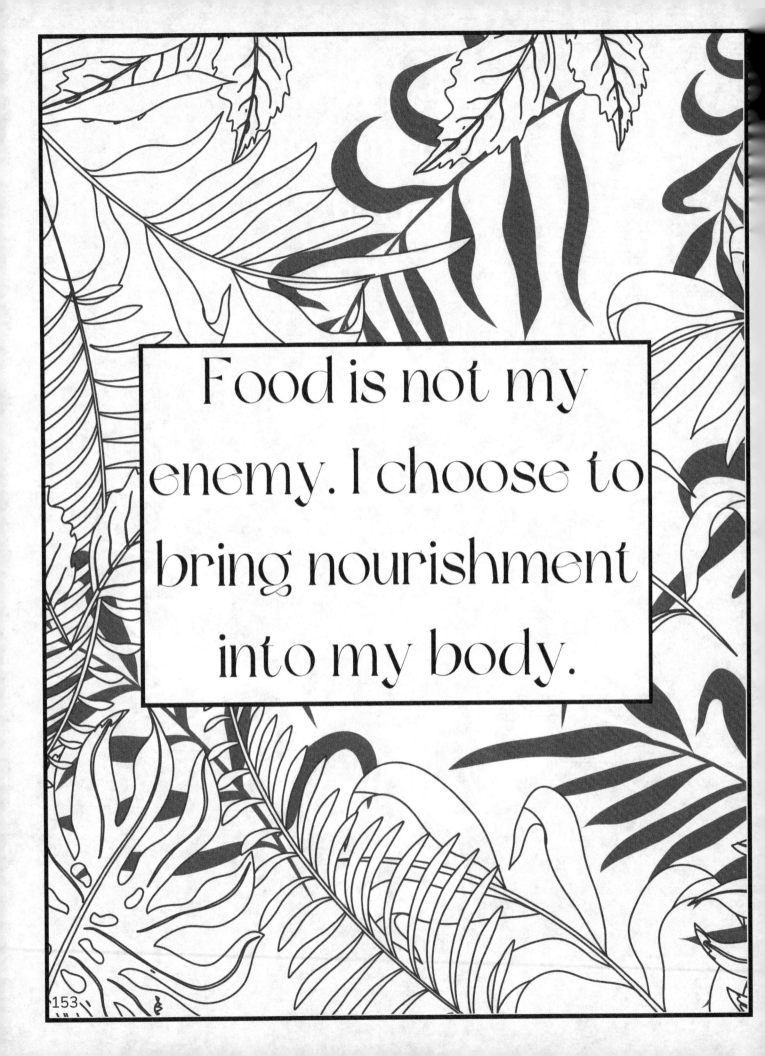

Food is not my enemy. I choose to bring nourishment into my body.

Now is the only time there is.

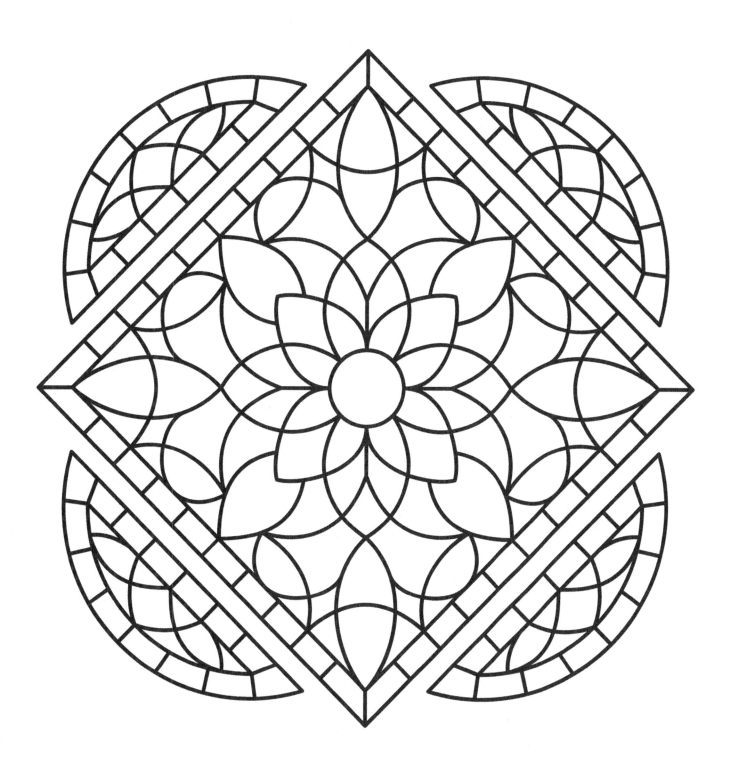

I can finally see, there is nothing wrong with me.

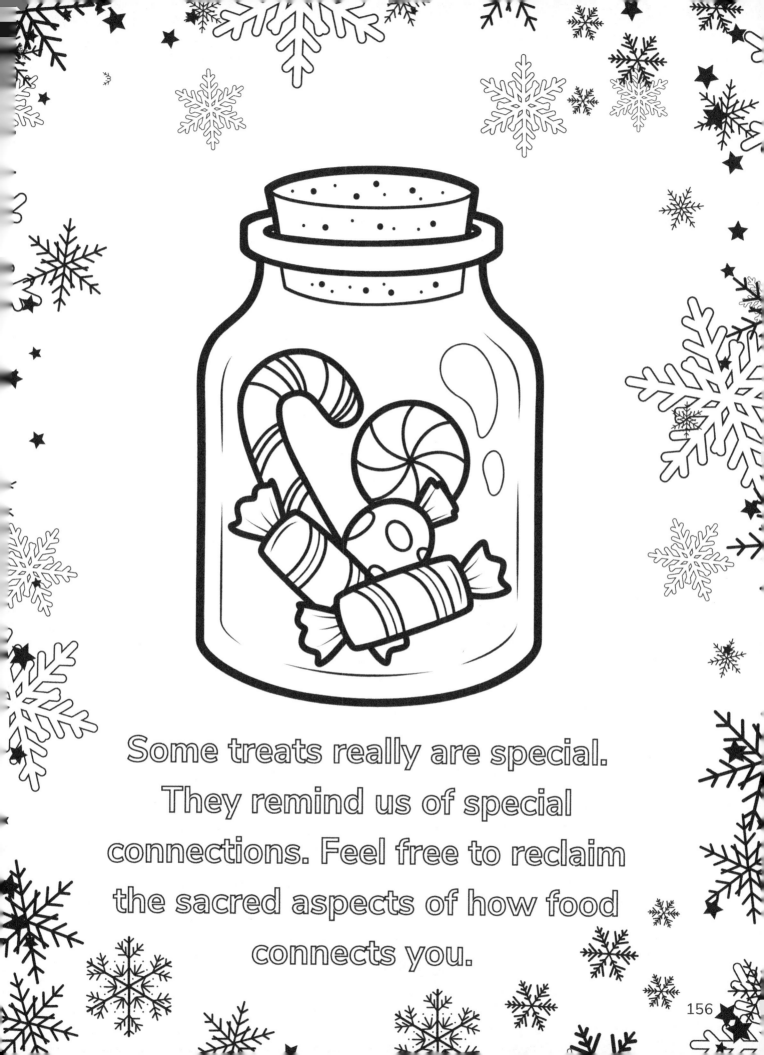

Some treats really are special. They remind us of special connections. Feel free to reclaim the sacred aspects of how food connects you.

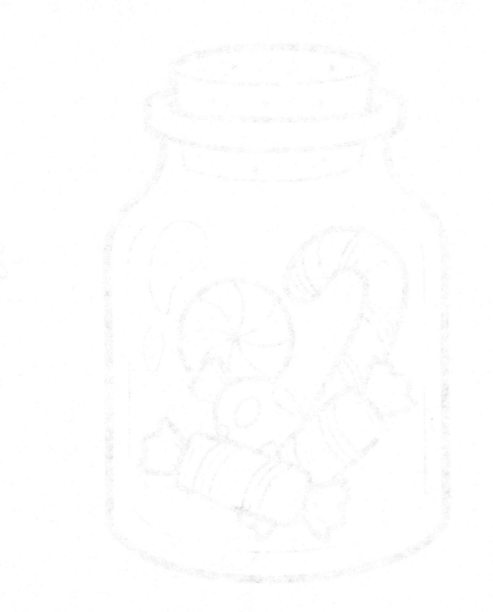

WHAT ARE YOUR SPECIAL FOODS? CAN YOU EAT THEM WITH REVERENCE?

This Page Intentionally Left Blank

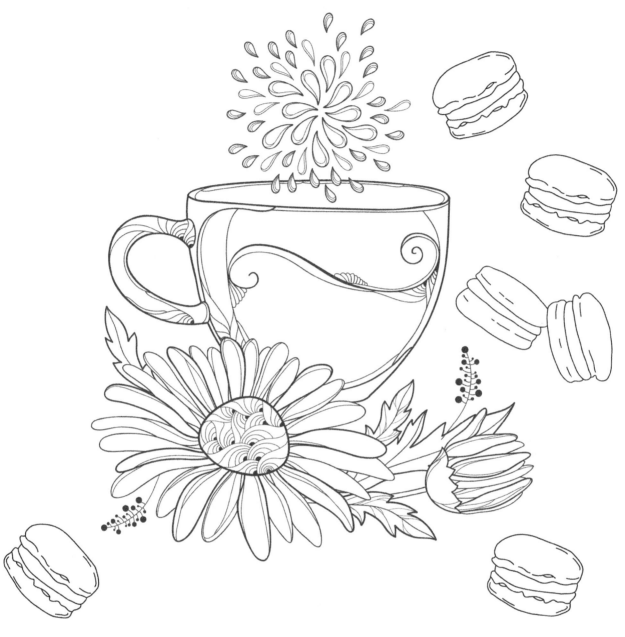

You set the rules now, you are an
adult, you do not have to prove you
deserve it. Pleasure is not a reward,
it is as natural as pain.

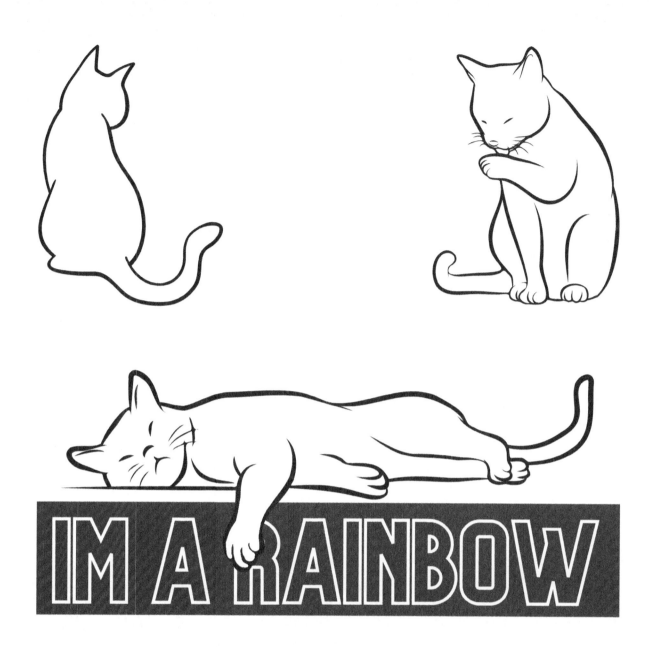

IM A RAINBOW

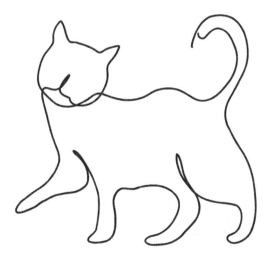

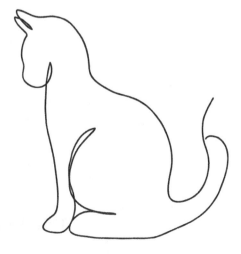

This Page Intentionally Left Blank

WHAT ARE YOUR COLORS? WHAT MAKES YOU LIGHT UP?

This Page Intentionally Left Blank

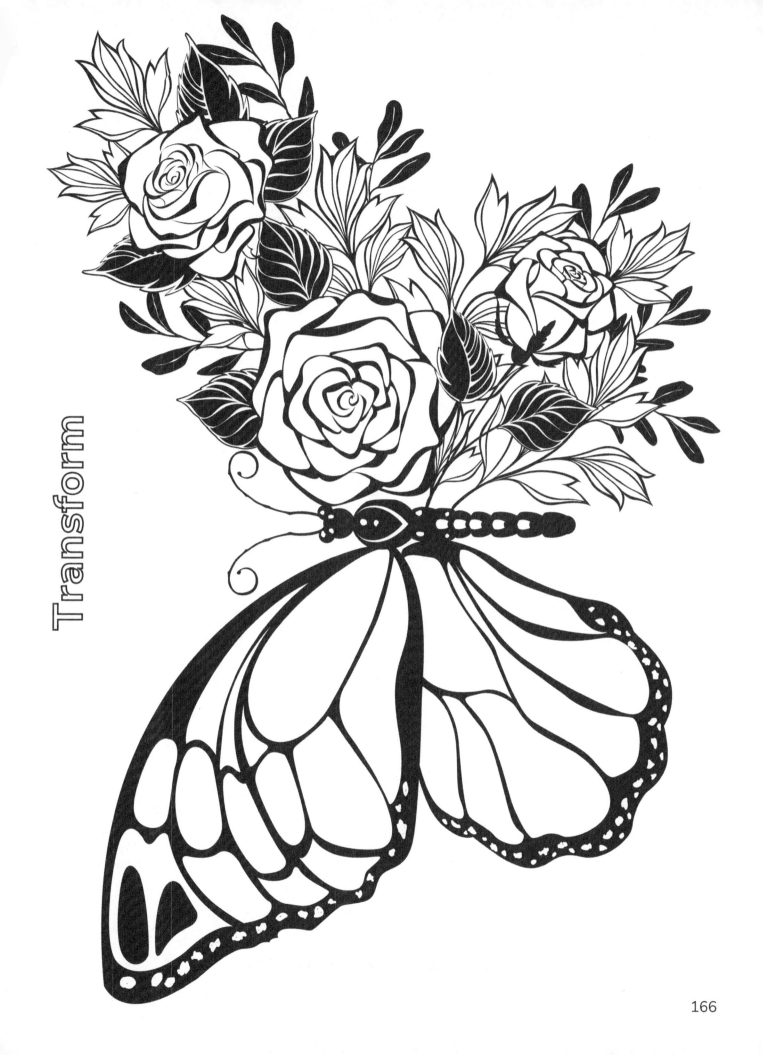

Transform

This Page Intentionally Left Blank

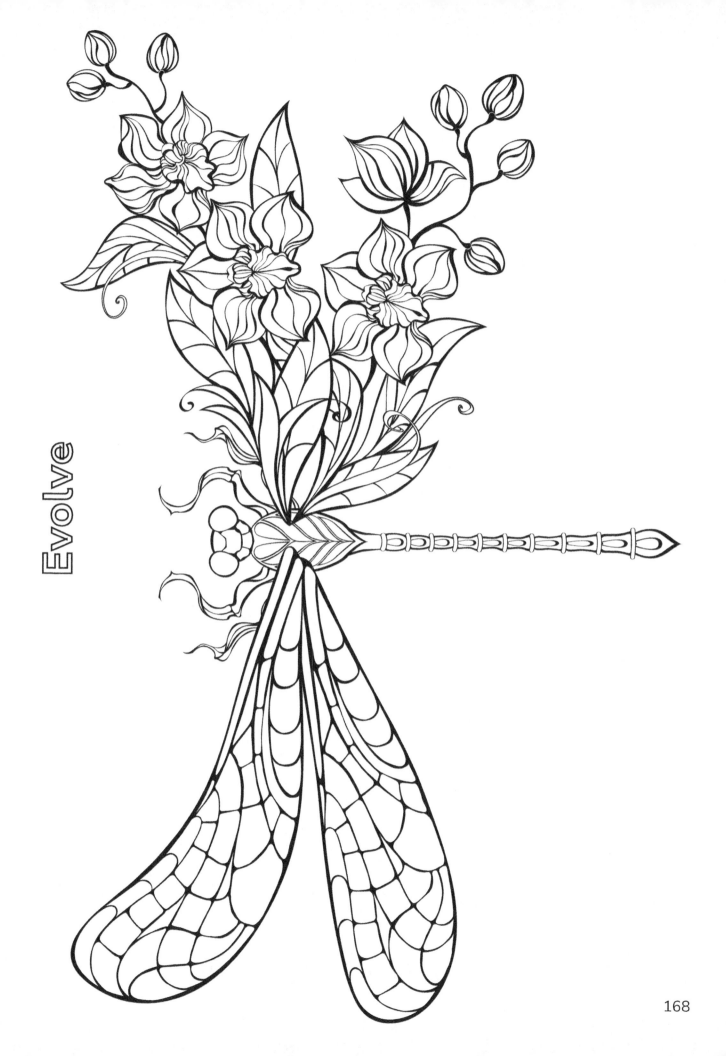

Evolve

This Page Intentionally Left Blank

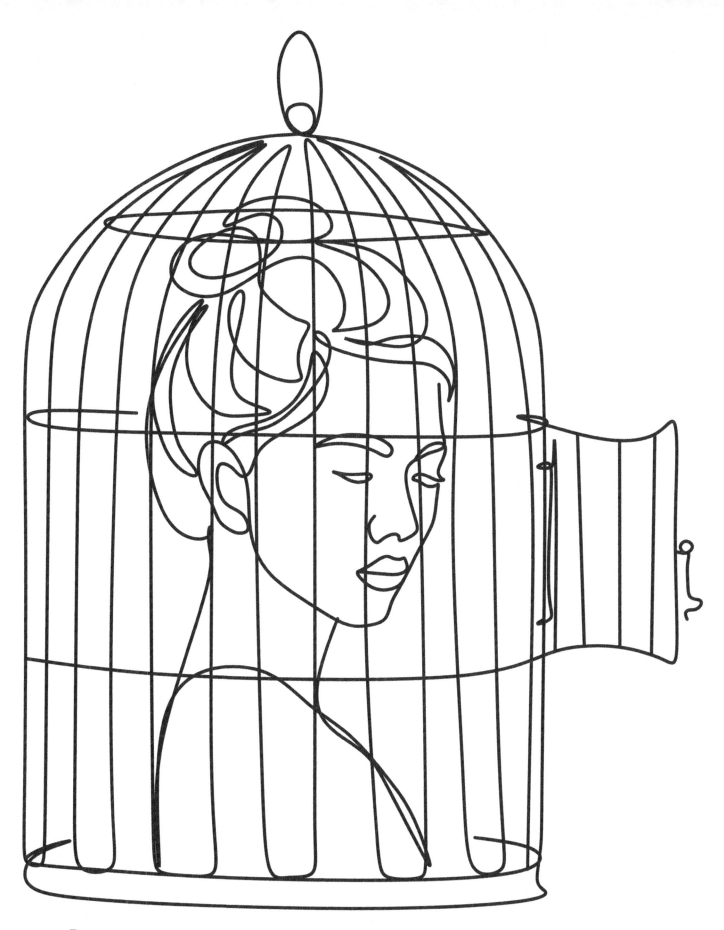

BELIEVE IN YOURSELF AND DON'T LET ANYONE TAKE
YOUR CONFIDENCE.

This Page Intentionally Left Blank

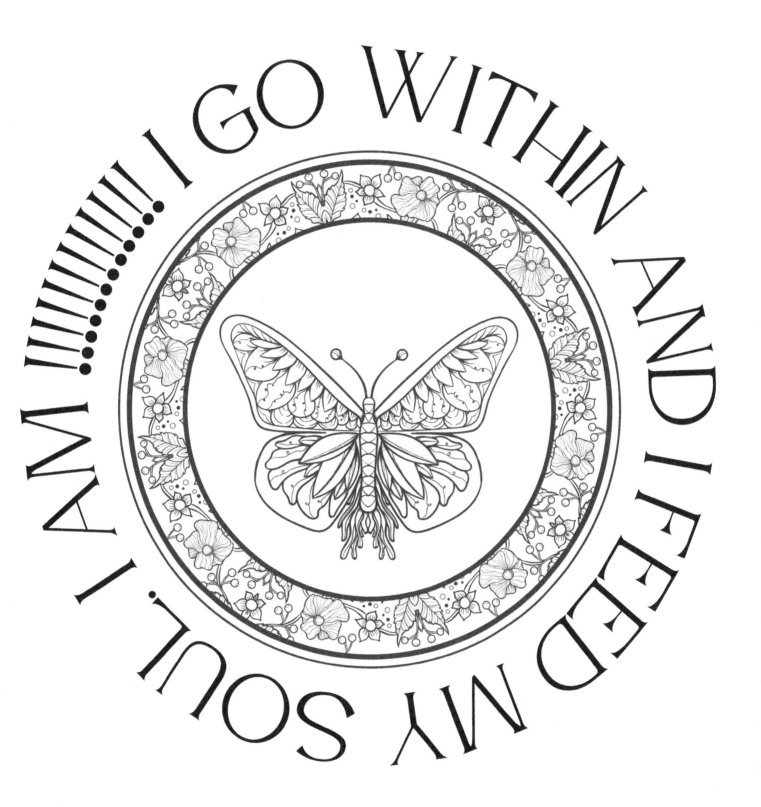

I GO WITHIN AND I FEED MY SOUL, I AM I AM

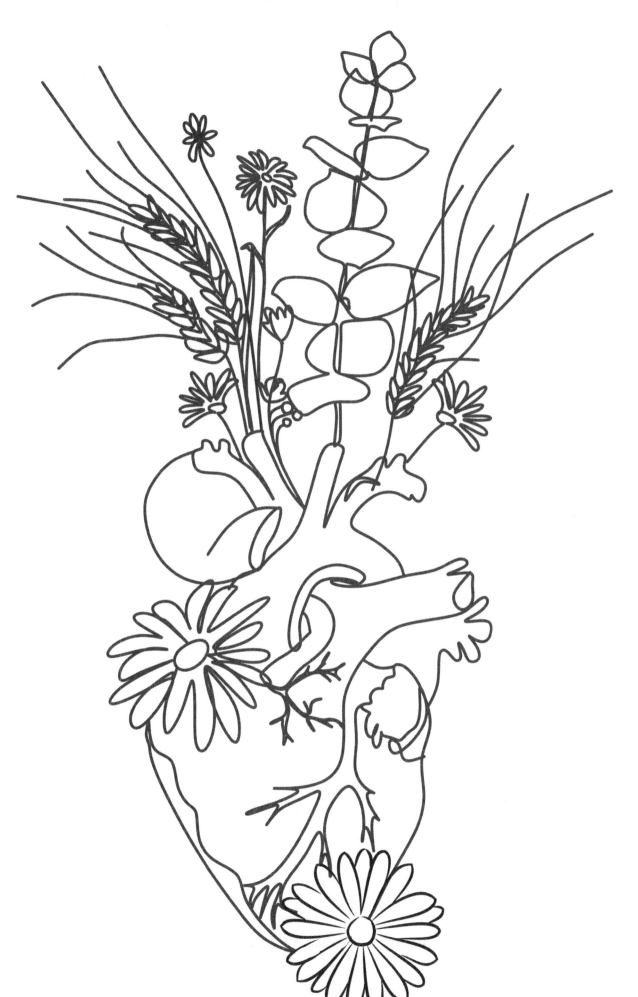

This Page Intentionally Left Blank

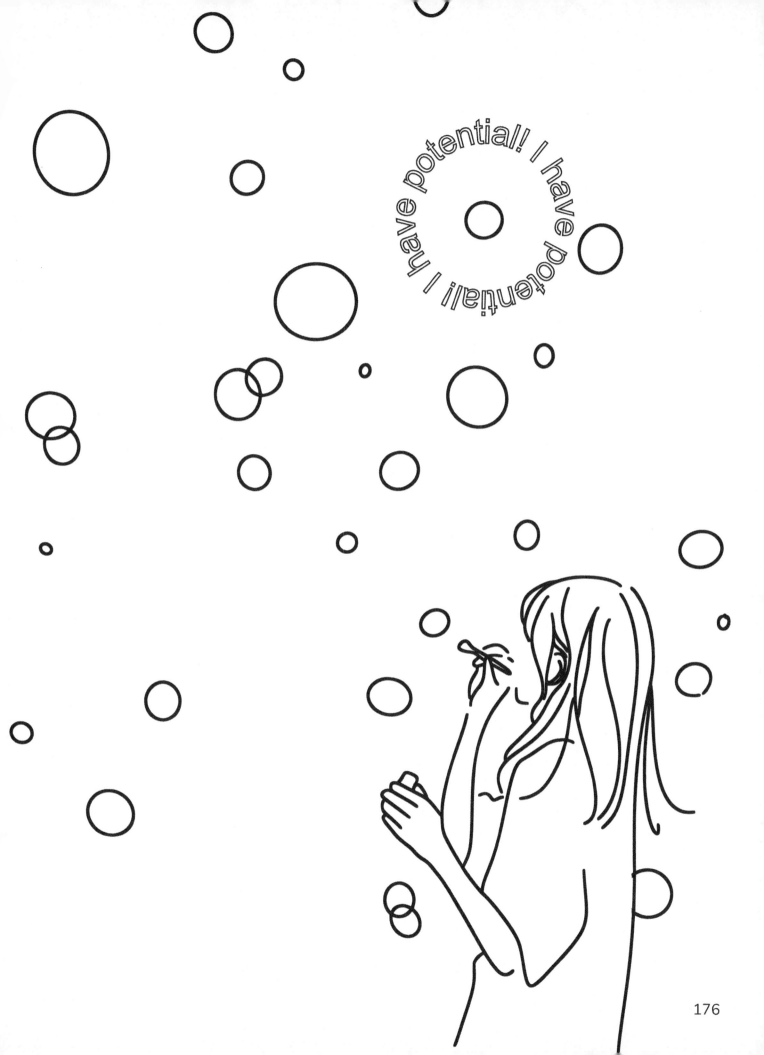

This Page Intentionally Left Blank

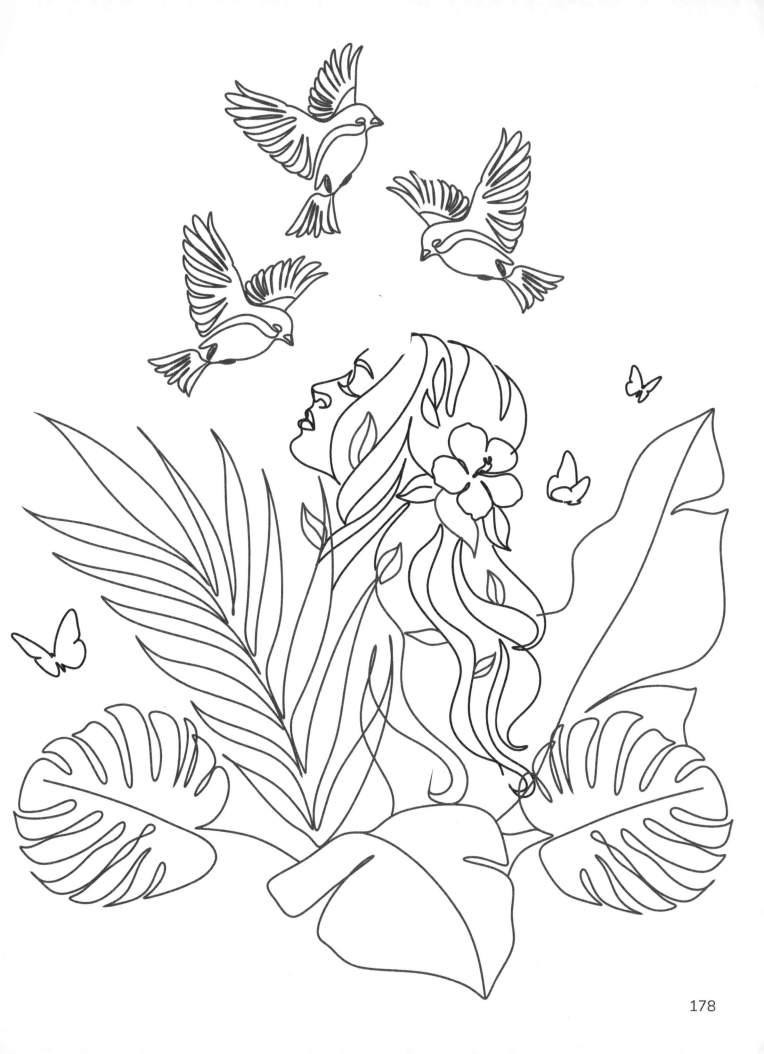

This Page Intentionally Left Blank

Imagine what it would take to have a life worth living. Could you still have a life worth living and make some compromises about what or how you eat?

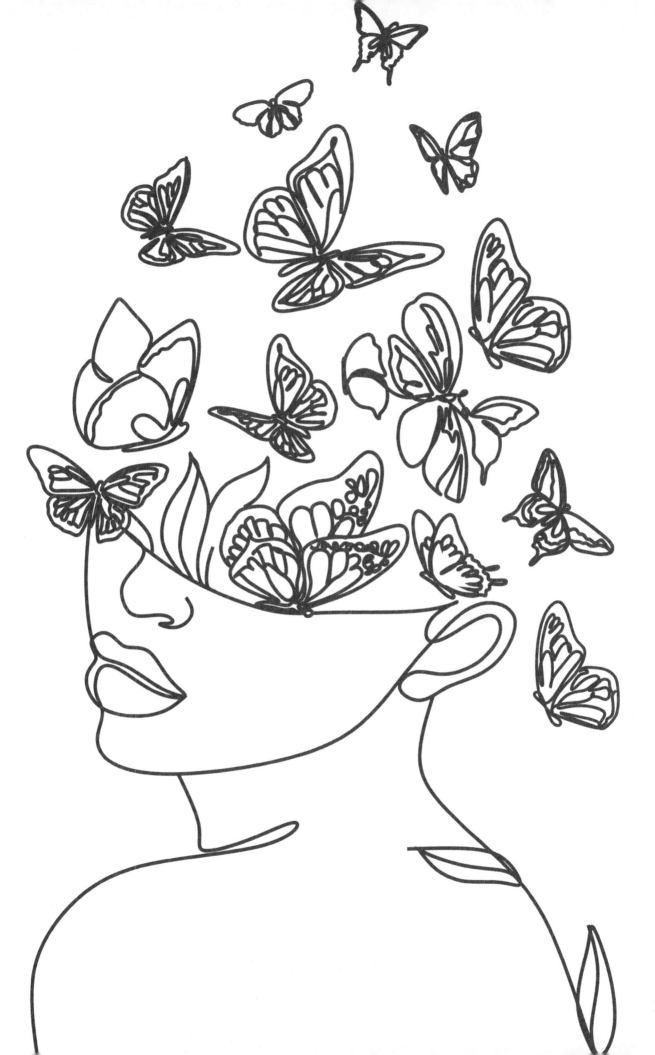

This Page Intentionally Left Blank

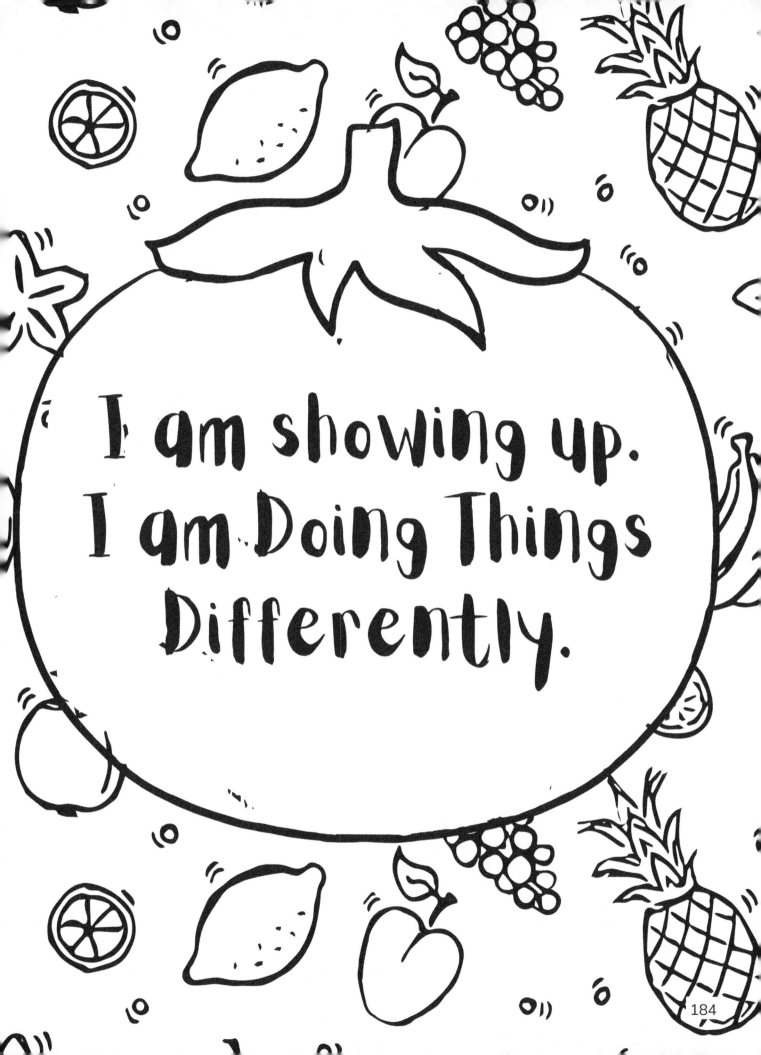

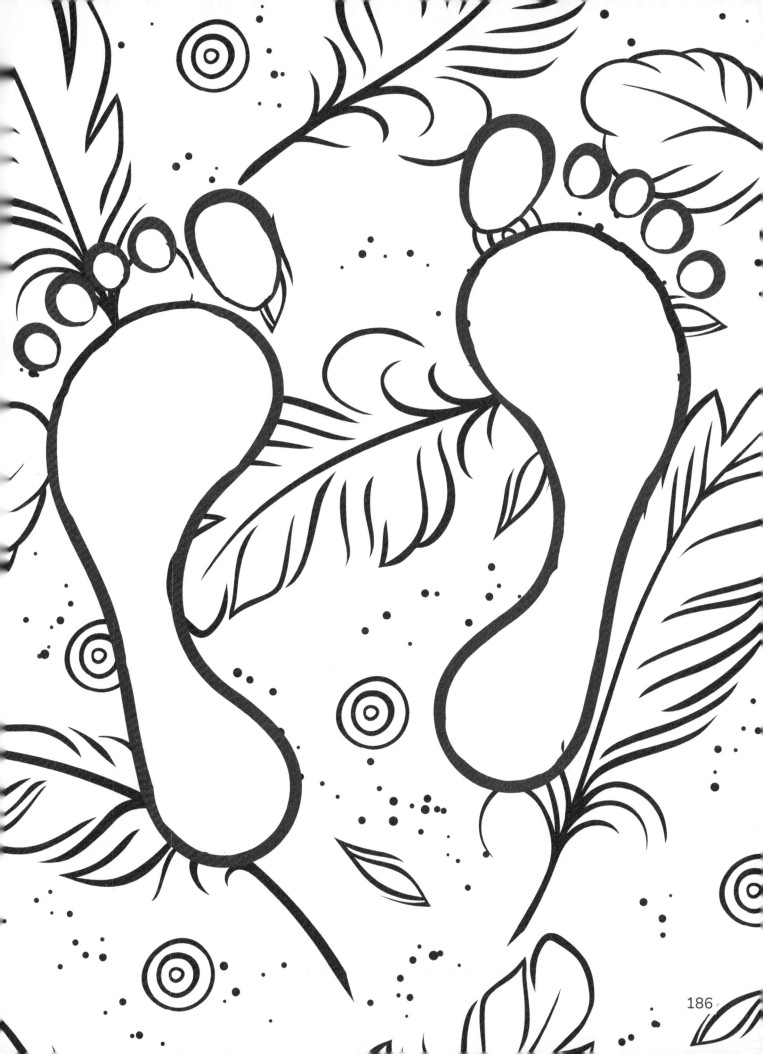

This Page Intentionally Left Blank

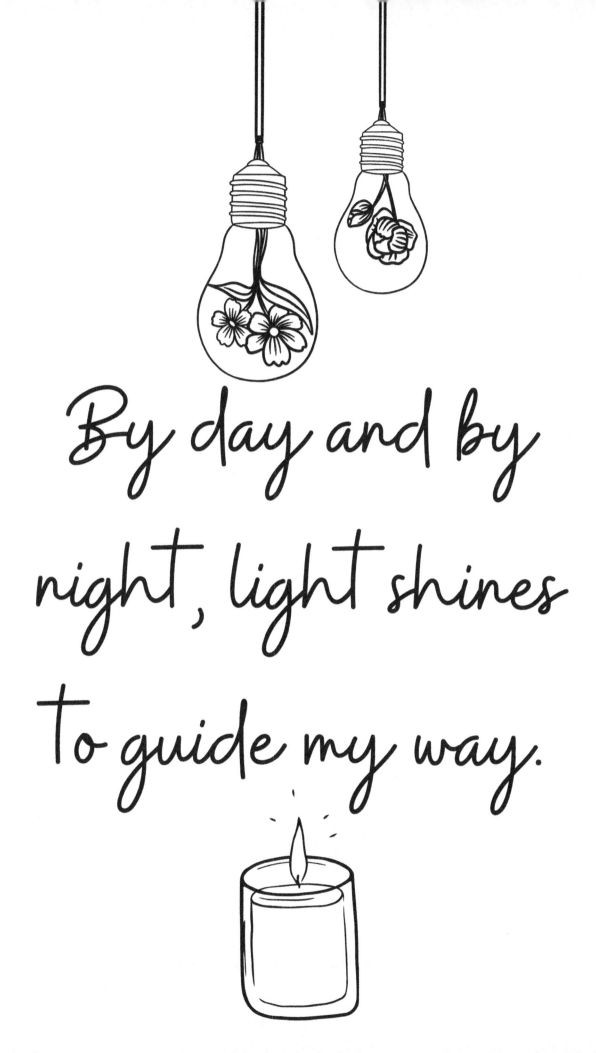

By day and by night, light shines to guide my way.

This Page Intentionally Left Blank

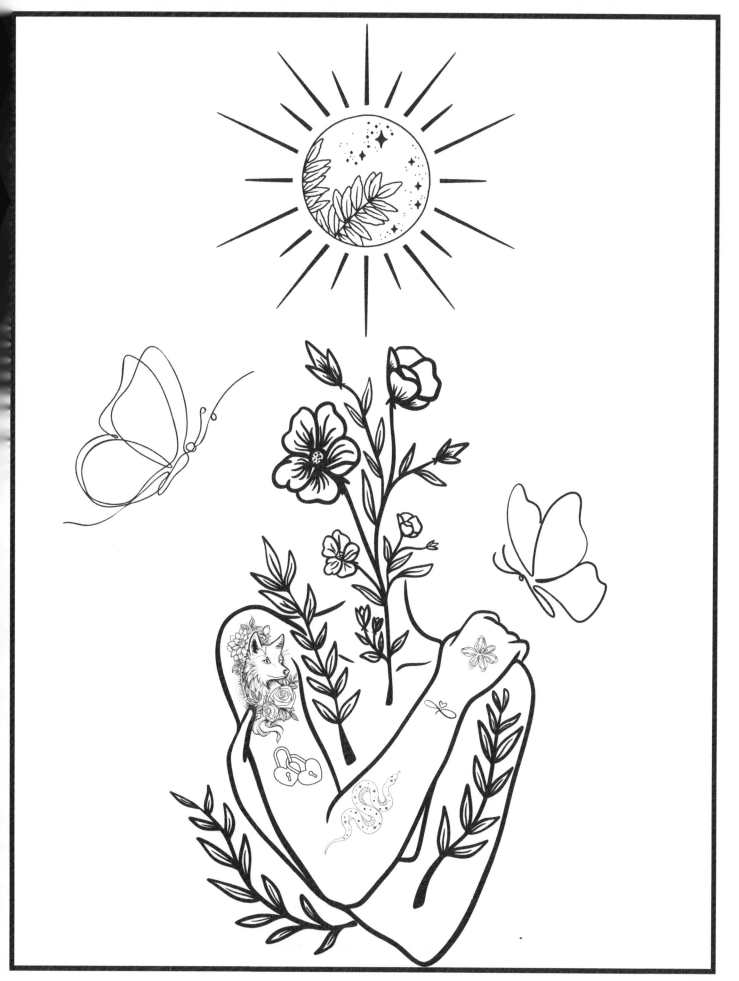

WHEN I AM EMPTY, IN ORDER TO FILL UP, I?

This Page Intentionally Left Blank

When
we resist
change,
it is
called
suffering
-Pema
Chodron

This Page Intentionally Left Blank

I am suffering because...

"I have so much self acceptance."
-Emily Atack

My Super Self Portrait!

This Page Intentionally Left Blank

Where once
there was only
darkness, now
light shines from
all of my cracks.
We are never
broken!

This Page Intentionally Left Blank

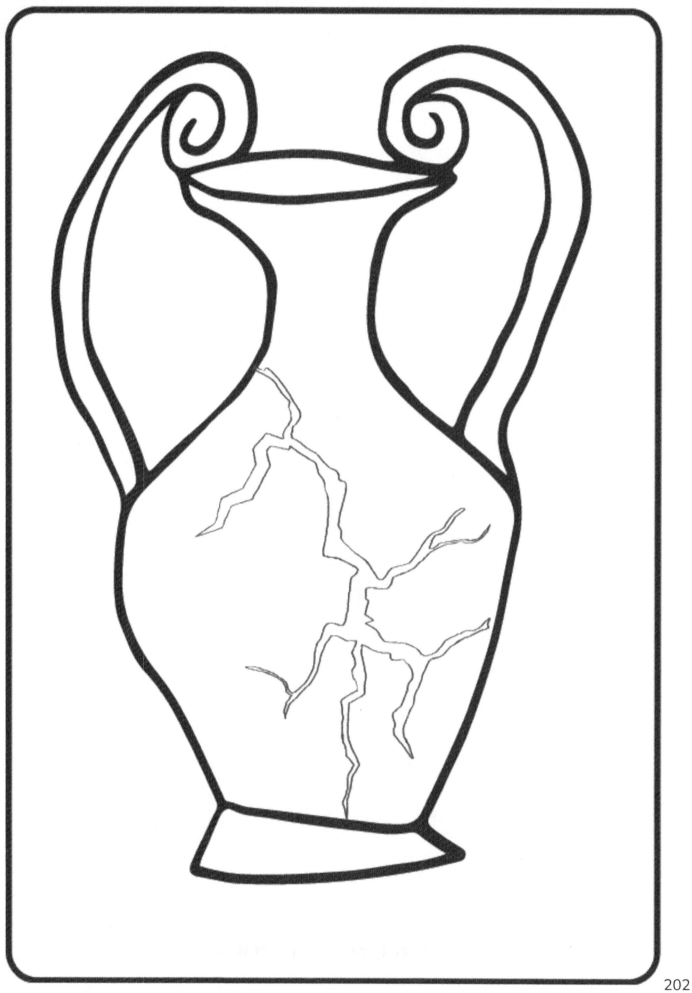

I trust my inner knowing and love myself.
I eat in a way that respects my body.

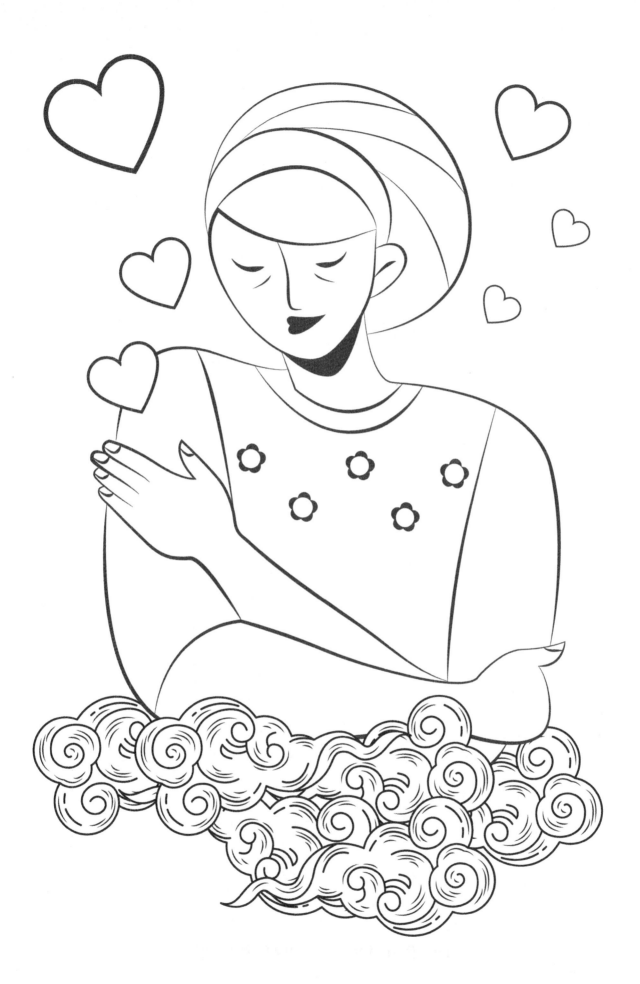

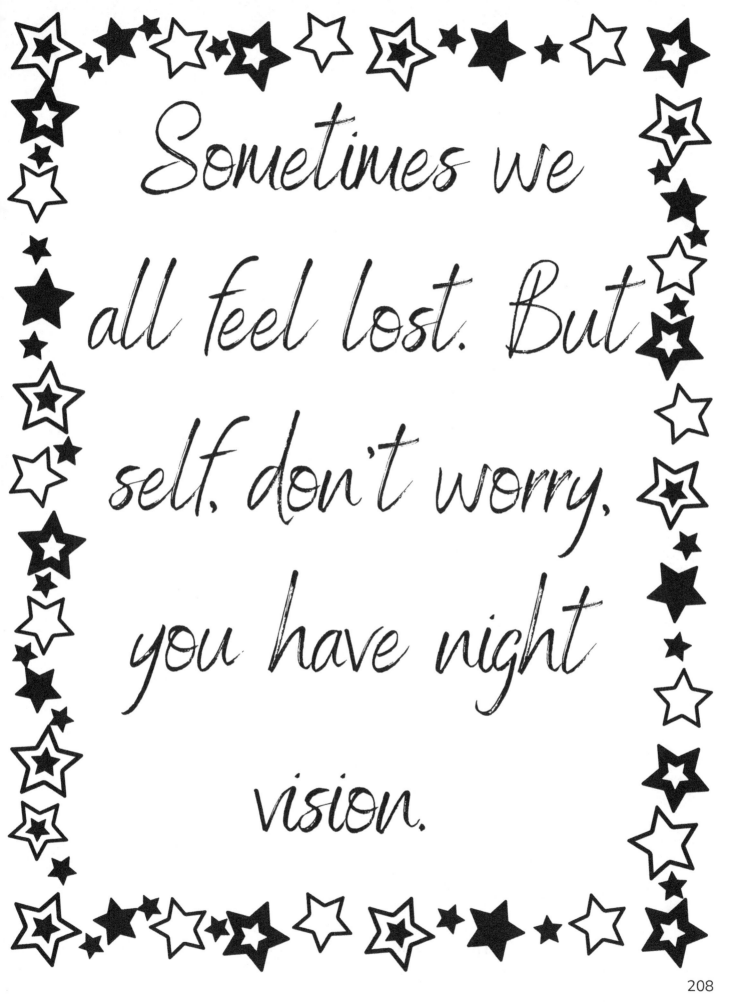

Sometimes we all feel lost. But self, don't worry, you have night vision.

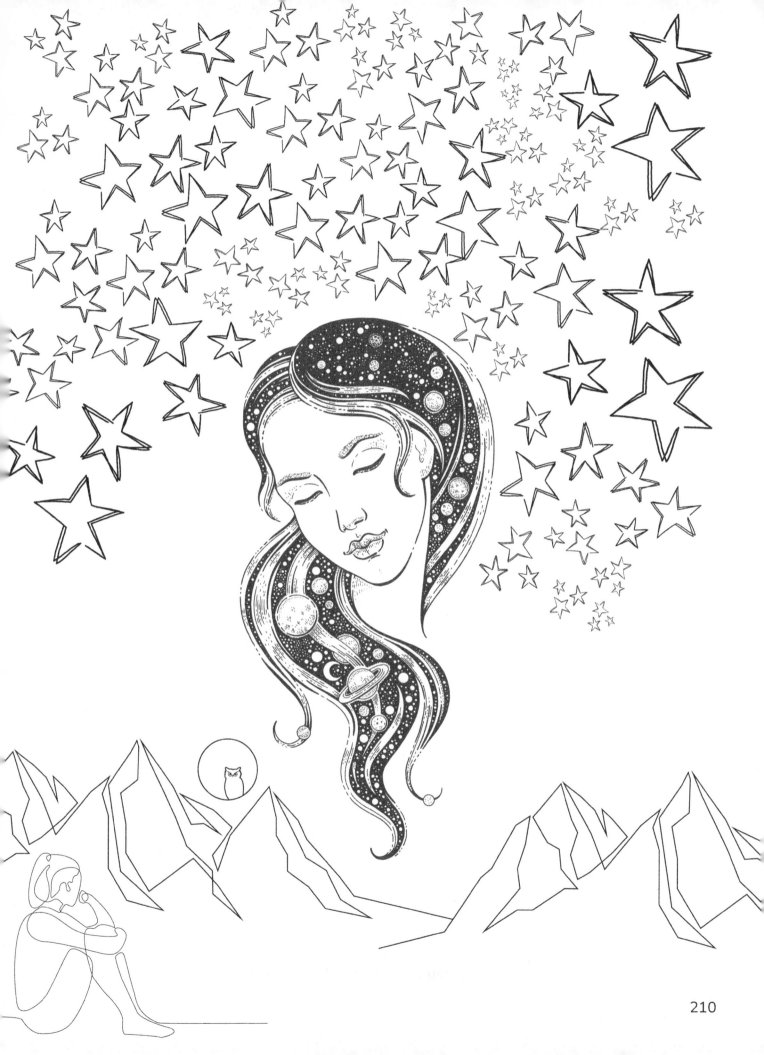

This Page Intentionally Left Blank

I AM CAPABLE OF SAYING BOTH

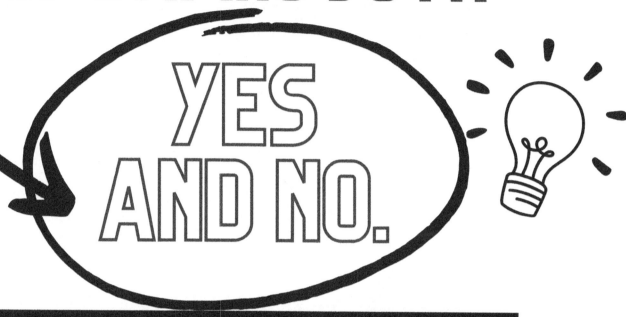

YES AND NO.

I have choices.

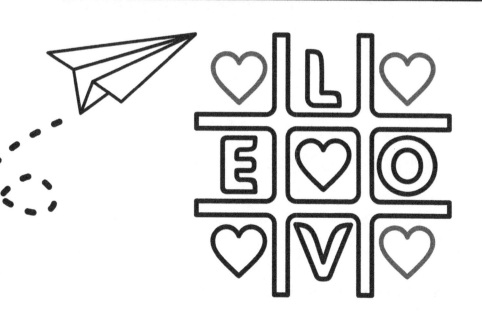

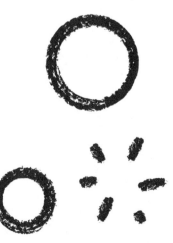

This Page Intentionally Left Blank

This Page Intentionally Left Blank

My child, there is a
sanctuary inside of
you.

-Your Inner Parent

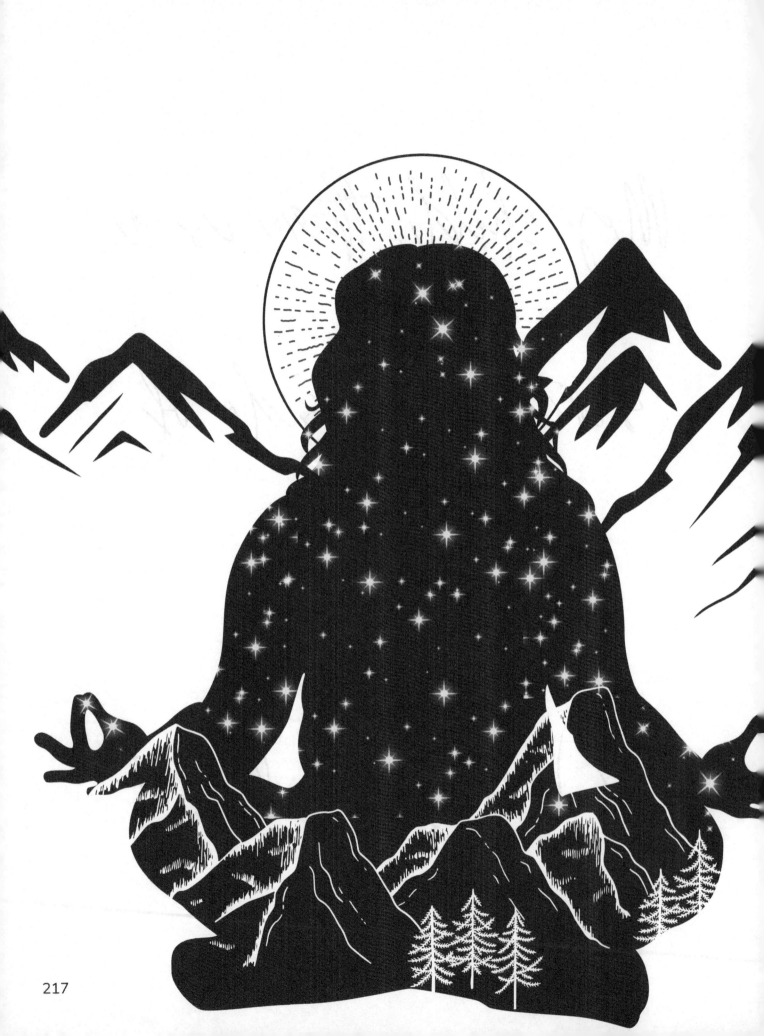

Relapse happens. What can I do to be a warrior for my health instead of a worrier about my health?

This Page Intentionally Left Blank

I appreciate food and what it provides my cells.
Make a list of some of the health benefits you
receive from food.

This Page Intentionally Left Blank

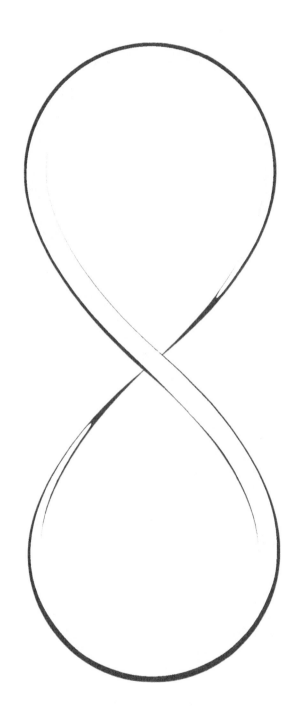

Quiet your mind, beloved one.

Trace the infinity shape, over and over, while inhaling and
exhaling at a slow and easy pace.

This Page Intentionally Left Blank

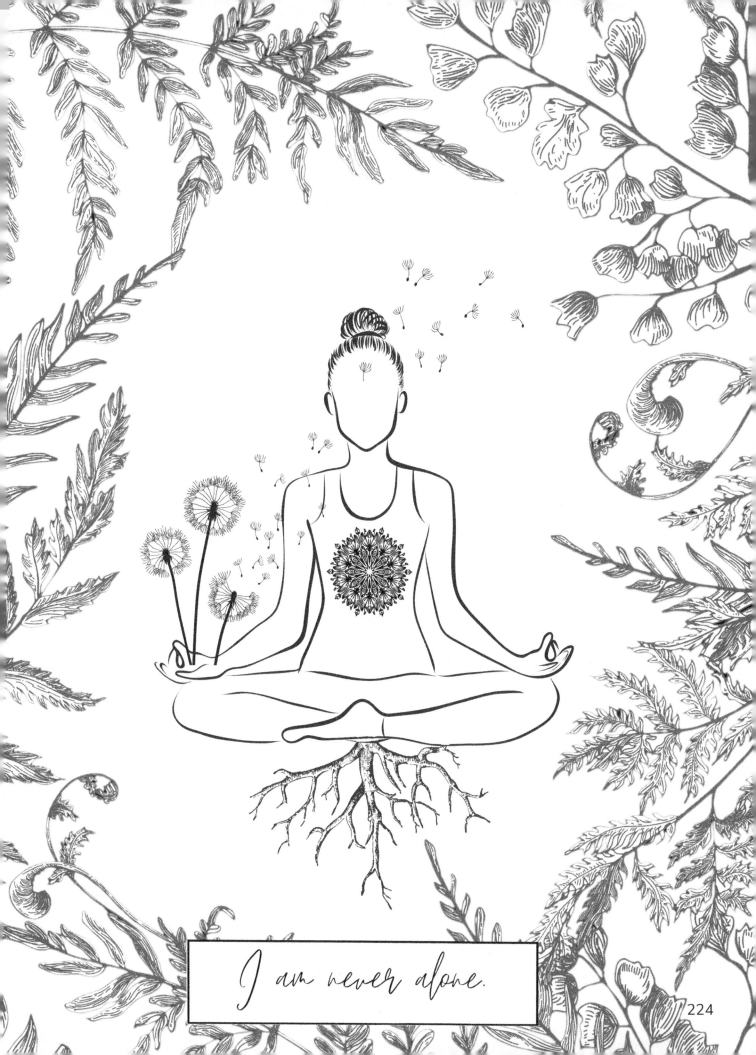

I am never alone.

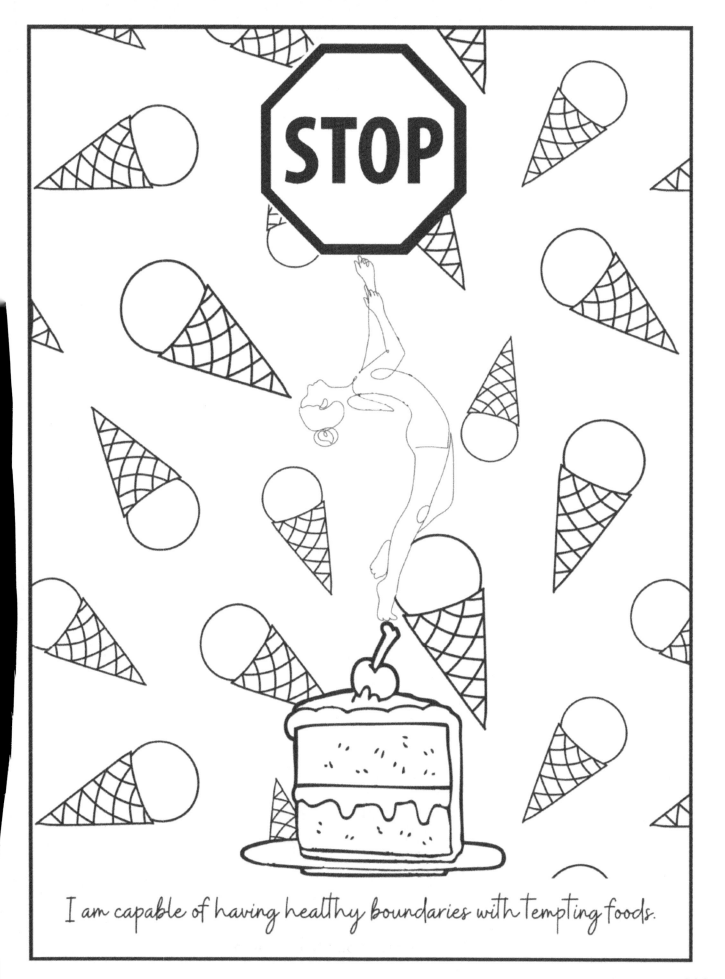

I am capable of having healthy boundaries with tempting foods.

Spend some time reflecting on what you have learned and how you have grown through the use of this activity book.

_____

_____

_____

_____

_____

_____

_____

_____

_____

_____

_____

_____

_____

References

Part I

1. Anguah, K. et al. (2019) 'Changes in food cravings and eating behavior after a dietary carbohydrate restriction intervention trial', Nutrients, 12(1), p. 52. doi:10.3390/nu12010052.

2. Augustine, V., Lee, S. and Oka, Y. (2020) 'Neural control and modulation of thirst, sodium appetite, and hunger', Cell, 180(1), pp. 25–32. doi:10.1016/j.cell.2019.11.040.

3. Borgna-Pignatti, C. and Zanella, S. (2016) 'Pica as a manifestation of iron deficiency', Expert Review of Hematology, 9(11), pp. 1075–1080. doi:10.1080/17474086.2016.1245136.

4. Cooper, E. (2015) The metabolic storm: The science of your metabolism and why it's making you fat and possibly infertile: P.S. it's not your fault. Seattle, WA: Seattle Performance Medicine.

5. DiNicolantonio, J.J. and Berger, A. (2016) 'Added sugars drive nutrient and energy deficit in obesity: A new paradigm', Open Heart, 3(2). doi:10.1136/openhrt-2016-000469.

6. Frederick, E. (2019) 'Why skimping on sleep makes your brain crave sweets', Science [Preprint]. doi:10.1126/science.aaz8839.

7. Gasmi, A. et al. (2022) 'Neurotransmitters regulation and food intake: The role of dietary sources in neurotransmission', Molecules, 28(1), p. 210. doi:10.3390/molecules28010210.

8. Greer, S.M., Goldstein, A.N. and Walker, M.P. (2013) 'The impact of sleep deprivation on food desire in the human brain', Nature Communications, 4(1). doi:10.1038/ncomms3259.

9. Gudipally, P.R. (2023) Premenstrual syndrome, StatPearls [Internet]. Available at: https://www.ncbi.nlm.nih.gov/books/NBK560698/ (Accessed: 19 April 2024).

10. Harington, K. et al. (2016) 'Desire for sweet taste unchanged after eating: Evidence of a dessert mentality?', Journal of the American College of Nutrition, 35(6), pp. 581–586. doi:10.1080/07315724.2015.1117956.

11. Hurley, S.W. and Johnson, A.K. (2015) 'The biopsychology of salt hunger and sodium deficiency', Pflügers Archiv - European Journal of Physiology, 467(3), pp. 445–456. doi:10.1007/s00424-014-1676-y.

12. Meule, A. (2020) 'The Psychology of Food Cravings: The role of food deprivation', Current Nutrition Reports, 9(3), pp. 251–257. doi:10.1007/s13668-020-00326-0.

13. Morris, M.J., Na, E.S. and Johnson, A.K. (2008) 'Salt craving: The psychobiology of pathogenic sodium intake', Physiology & Behavior, 94(5), pp. 709–721. doi:10.1016/j.physbeh.2008.04.008.

14. Nechifor, M. (2018) 'Magnesium in addiction – a general view', Magnesium Research, 31(3), pp. 90–98. doi:10.1684/mrh.2018.0443.

15. Rodin, J. (1985) 'Insulin levels, hunger, and food intake: An example of feedback loops in body weight regulation.', Health Psychology, 4(1), pp. 1–24. doi:10.1037//0278-6133.4.1.1.

16. Sun, W. and Kober, H. (2020) 'Regulating food craving: From mechanisms to interventions', Physiology & Behavior, 222, p. 112878. doi:10.1016/j.physbeh.2020.112878.

17. Understanding PMS and your cycle (no date) Saint Luke's Health System. Available at: https://www.saintlukeskc.org/health-library/understanding-pms-and-your-cycle#:~:text=The%20PMS%20cycle&text=Estrogen%20rises%20during%20the%20first,2%20weeks%20before%20the%20period. (Accessed: 19 April 2024).

18. Wansink, B. (2011) Mindless eating. Hay House UK Ltd.

19. Trevelline, B. K., & Kohl, K. D. (2022). The gut microbiome influences host diet selection behavior. Proceedings of the National Academy of Sciences of the United States of America, 119(17). https://doi.org/10.1073/pnas.2117537119

20. Ousey, J., Boktor, J. C., & Mazmanian, S. K. (2023). Gut microbiota suppress feeding induced by palatable foods. In Current Biology (Vol. 33, Issue 1, pp. 147-157.e7). Elsevier BV. https://doi.org/10.1016/j.cub.2022.10.066

21. Cronin P, Joyce SA, O'Toole PW, et al. Dietary Fibre Modulates the Gut Microbiota. Nutrients. May 13, 2021.

References

22. De Almeida, R., Kamath, G., & Cabandugama, P. (2022). Food addiction in application to Obesity Management. Missouri medicine. https://www.ncbi.nlm.nih.gov/pmc/articles/PMC9462897/

23. Penzenstadler, L., Khazaal, L., Karila, L., & Soares , C. (n.d.). Systematic review of food addiction as measured with the Yale Food Addiction Scale: Implications for the Food Addiction construct. Current neuropharmacology. https://pubmed.ncbi.nlm.nih.gov/30406740/

Part II

1. 3 quick DBT skills to help regulate anxiety that anyone can use! (no date) 3 Quick DBT Skills to Help Regulate Anxiety That Anyone Can Use!: Intrepid Mental Wellness, PLLC: Psychiatric Nurse Practitioners. Available at: https://www.intrepidmentalhealth.com/blog/3-quick-dbt-skills-to-help-regulate-anxiety-that-anyone-can-use (Accessed: 19 April 2024).

2. Bays, J.C. (2017) Mindful eating a guide to rediscovering a healthy and joyful relationship with food. Boston: Shambhala.

3. Cognitive distortions: Unhelpful thinking habits (2023) Psychology Tools. Available at: https://www.psychologytools.com/articles/unhelpful-thinking-styles-cognitive-distortions-in-cbt/ (Accessed: 19 April 2024).

4. Linehan, M. (2015) DBT skills training handouts and worksheets. New York: The Guilford Press.

5. M;, H.Y. (no date) [chewing and cognitive function], Brain and nerve = Shinkei kenkyu no shinpo. Available at: https://pubmed.ncbi.nlm.nih.gov/24371128/#:~:text=Chewing%20does%20not%20only%20crush,including%20alertness%20and%20executive%20function. (Accessed: 19 April 2024).

6. Spoor, S.T.P. et al. (2007) 'Relations between negative affect, coping, and emotional eating', Appetite, 48(3), pp. 368–376. doi:10.1016/j.appet.2006.10.005.

Part III

1. Cordero RDN, L.L. (2021) The 5D's: Cravings and Taming Your Inner Beast, Nourish2Thrive. Available at: https://nourish2thrive.net/5ds-cravings/ (Accessed: 19 April 2024).

2. Linehan, M. (2015) DBT skills training handouts and worksheets. New York: The Guilford Press.

3. Team, C.E. (2024) 5, 4, 3, 2, 1 - a simple grounding exercise to calm anxiety, Calm Blog. Available at: https://www.calm.com/blog/5-4-3-2-1-a-simple-exercise-to-calm-the-mind#:~:text=What%20is%20the%2054321%20method,1%20thing%20you%20can%20taste. (Accessed: 19 April 2024).

Made in the USA
Monee, IL
14 November 2024

70056392R00129